THE MISSING
WELLNESS
FACTORS—
EPA AND DHA

THE MISSING WELLNESS FACTORS— EPA AND DHA

The Most Important Nutrients Since Vitamins?

JØRN DYERBERG, M.D., DMSc. &
RICHARD A. PASSWATER, PH.D.

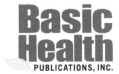

Basic Health PUBLICATIONS, INC.

Basic Health Publications, Inc.
www.basichealthpub.com

Library of Congress Cataloging-in-Publication Data

Dyerberg, Jørn.
　　The missing wellness factors : EPA and DHA the most important nutrients since vitamins? / Jørn Dyerberg and Richard A. Passwater.
　　　p. cm.
　　Includes bibliographical references and index.
　　ISBN 978-1-59120-300-1 Paperback
　　ISBN 978-1-68162-630-7 Hardback
　1. Eicosanoids—Therapeutic use. 2. Docosahexaenoic acid—Health aspects. 3. Omega-3 fatty acids—Health aspects. I. Passwater, Richard A. II. Title.
　　QP752.E53D94　　2012
　　612'.01577—dc23

                                                    2012019065

Editor: Cheryl Hirsch
Copyeditor: Susan E. Davis
Typesetting/Book design: Gary A. Rosenberg
Cover design: Mike Stromberg
Diagrams and photos: Jørn Dyerberg, M.D., DMSc., and Richard A. Passwater, Ph.D.

Printed in the United States of America

10　9　8　7　6　5　4　3　2

Contents

Foreword

Most doctors recommend omega-3 supplements, typically from fish oil, to all their patients. Why? One reason is that in the United States about 84,000 deaths per year are attributable to low intake of these essential oils. People with higher blood levels of omega-3 have been shown to be 90 percent less likely to develop sudden cardiac arrest than those with low (normal) levels. What's more, in one large study, heart patients given omega-3 capsules cut their risk of sudden death nearly in half. Remarkably, a similar story is developing for Alzheimer's disease where people with the highest omega-3 levels were about 50 percent less likely to develop dementia over nine years. Since there is no known health risk from taking omega-3 supplements, it is my view that virtually every American should either eat more omega-3 rich fish (salmon, sardines, mackerel, herring, albacore tuna, etc.) or take fish oil (EPA/DHA) supplements.

This book explains how fish oil provides you with many health benefits and guides you to adopt optimal usage of the essential nutrients found in fish oil. All that you need to know about fish oil—from the initial discovery in Greenland of how it protects against heart disease to the latest research on how it reduces the risk of Alzheimer's disease—has been distilled from thousands of scientific studies and hundreds of clinical trials and condensed into practical information you can use to improve your health now and to live better longer.

I don't know of anybody who would not benefit from learning more about fish oil and its many health advantages, which range from preventing heart disease, arthritis, diabetes, and dementias to staying younger longer. Jørn Dyerberg, M.D., DMSc., is the primary discoverer of the role of fish oil in preventing heart disease and of how the nutrients in fish oils are essential to optimal health. Until now, Dr. Dyerberg has published this information only in technical articles that don't reach the majority of people. Thankfully, the well-respected health writer and antioxidant researcher Richard Passwater, Ph.D., (who wrote the very first book on fish oil and preventing heart disease) has now coaxed the fascinating story out of the modest, unassuming Dr. Dyerberg.

Dr. Passwater, who first learned of Dr. Dyerberg's seminal research in 1981, has published two books on fish oil (in 1982 and 1987), but many more exciting health benefits have been discovered since then. As the two colleagues shared information, Dr. Passwater convinced Dr. Dyerberg to tell his story for the benefit of all readers, not just the scientific community. This is not boasting or bragging; it is simply recounting the historic series of observations and scientific discoveries that even Dr. Dyerberg could not imagine would have ensued from his explorations along the frozen coastline of Greenland over four decades ago. His initial findings ultimately resulted in new insights that are now saving lives every day.

I am personally indebted to the pioneering research of Dr. Dyerberg for shaping my professional career. Back in 1979, when I was a post-doctoral fellow at the Oregon Health Sciences University (Portland), I worked in the lab of Dr. William Connor, a giant in the study of nutrition, lipids, and heart disease. My assignment was to design and carry out a study on the effects on blood cholesterol levels of a diet very high in salmon oil (about 100 grams per day!). We were unaware at that time of the work of Drs. Dyerberg and Bang in Greenland, which pinpointed the omega-3 fatty acids as the cardioprotective factors in the Eskimos' diet; we were simply interested in the overall "polyunsaturated-ness" of fish oil. Would it *lower* cholesterol like other liquid oils (which were plant-not animal-derived)? Or would it *raise* cholesterol like other animal fats (which were solid not liquid)? We did find that the "liquid-ness" was more important than the "animal-ness" of the oil vis-à-vis blood cholesterol, but when we learned about omega-3 fatty acids from Drs. Dyerberg and Bang, our blinders fell off and we began to see fish oils not simply as liquid animal fats, but as vehicles for terribly important nutrients—ones that were sadly missing from the American diet.

That shift in focus has guided my research over the last thirty years, to the point where we now believe that the blood omega-3 level ("the omega-3 index") is actually a heart disease *risk factor*—a marker in the blood that predicts risk for fatal heart attacks (and probably other maladies) that, importantly, can be changed by altering the diet. I believe the omega-3 index is even more important than the cholesterol level when it comes to identifying patients at increased risk for heart attacks. As of this writing, the omega-3 index has formally entered the world of medical care and is being included in routine lipid panels at a major clinical lab (Health Diagnostic Laboratory, Richmond, Va.), and is helping hundreds of physicians manage cardiac risk for thousands of patients. Without the visionary work and tireless investigation of Dr. Dyerberg, the omega-3 index would not exist today.

I am thankful that these two highly qualified scientists—Drs. Dyerberg and Passwater—have joined forces to bring the omega-3 story to the general public. You will enjoy the adventure that awaits you in these pages, and if "you have ears to hear," you too can begin to enjoy the health benefits provided from these "gifts from the sea."

William S. Harris, Ph.D.
Sioux Falls, South Dakota
February 2012

Preface

Dr. Jørn Dyerberg's quest to find out why the high-fat diets of Eskimos resulted in less heart disease than the diets of their more Westernized brethren led to a serendipitous discovery that can help to protect many of us from heart disease. But, more importantly, Dr. Dyerberg's discovery has led to a new class of nutrients essential to all human health—more than just heart health!

Thanks to the research initiated by Dr. Dyerberg and his colleagues, we now know that the nutrients EPA (eicosapentaenoic acid) and DHA (docosahexaenoic acid) are required by the body for their unique vital functions. However, these omega-3 essential fatty acids are inadequate in modern diets and, furthermore, are continuing to disappear at an accelerated pace. Other nutrients, even of the same omega-3 family of fats, cannot perform the unique vital functions of EPA and DHA. These fatty acids are similar in many ways, but, as we will explain later, each has separate and independent functions. We must depend on our diets to provide adequate amounts of both EPA and DHA. Not just one or the other, but both.

While Western medicine was focusing on cholesterol and fats as the major cause of heart disease in the 1960s, the Eskimos were providing Dr. Dyerberg with a more important cause—and prevention—of heart disease and many other diseases and disorders.

In this book, we will travel with Dr. Dyerberg to Greenland as he and his colleagues unlock the clues to this health mystery that is proving to be the most important health discovery since vitamins. We will then look at the scientific research and many clinical studies that show the importance of this new class of nutrients to heart and artery health, to brain function and the prevention of dementias including Alzheimer's disease, and to the easing of arthritis and diabetes' symptoms, and to keeping every cell in our bodies young.

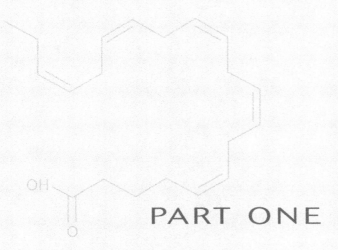

PART ONE

In the Beginning: The Discovery

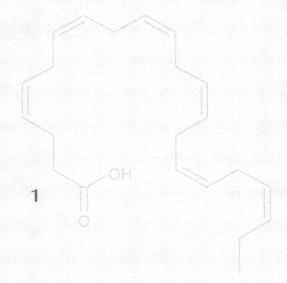

1

Unlocking the Eskimos' Nutritional Treasure

The yapping of the huskies was simmering down, but the biting Arctic wind still made conversation difficult. Dr. Jørn Dyerberg had many questions as the scientific expedition's eight dogsleds hauled by eighty-eight huskies glided over the sea ice (Figure 1.1). But he had to keep his thoughts to himself, as the only companion on his sled was the driver, Jonas, who only spoke Inuit. In fact, away from the towns, there were no noises other than the wind and whatever sounds you might be making. The quiet was striking.

Dr. Dyerberg and Dr. Hans Olaf "H.O." Bang were leading a Danish

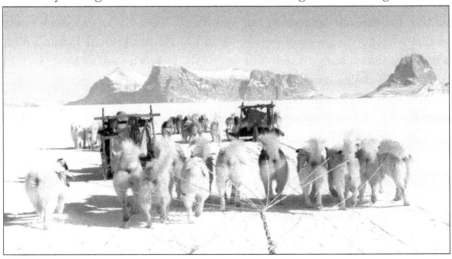

Figure 1.1. A view from the dogsled of Dr. Jørn Dyerberg on one of his expeditions to remote Greenland Inuit villages. The view never changes except for the lead dog.

3

research team in April 1972 to the settlement Igdlorssuit (now called Illorsuit) on Unknown Island, some eighty miles out from the coastline of northern Greenland in Baffin's Bay. At the settlement, approximately ninety Eskimos (Inuits) lived as hunters and fishers, in ways they had done for generations.

Let's pick up the story in Dr. Dyerberg's own words when they had been underway for ten hours, and both the dogs, dragging the heavy load of personal and scientific gear, and the passengers, unaccustomed to this type of traveling, were getting tired.

SCIENTIFIC ENDEAVOR AND PERSONAL ADVENTURE

I was wondering: Would this trip give us the final clue or are we on a wild goose chase? During our previous expedition in August–September 1970, we had uncovered some interesting clues, but we need a final piece of the puzzle to solve the mystery of why Eskimos don't have heart disease. We had found, in spite of their high fat diet, that the Eskimos had favorable cholesterol and blood lipid (fat) levels. Traveling and living far above the Arctic Circle wasn't what I had in mind when I joined Dr. Bang's research group, but it certainly gives room for experiences! Will our efforts be well received by the Eskimos? Will months of preparations that had brought us this far give an answer to our question? Now we are at least ready to test whether the answer will be found in the traditional Eskimo diet, which consists mainly of seal and fatty fish. It was a race against time as the world was changing, including the world of the Eskimo.

I thought to myself: We'll just have to start by collecting all the facts that we can. I hope my new blood analysis technique will help us. The daylong trip over the frozen sea under a sun that doesn't set has at least been an experience not many are given. As the team's technician said during a tea pause, "If not for the amount of clothes I am wearing, I would have pinched my arm to see if I was dreaming." Tea pauses were popular because they were warm, and tea could be made from melted ice so we didn't have to carry heavy water (Figure 1.2).

Flashback

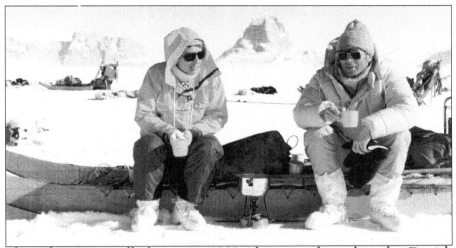

This adventure really began in 1968 when an editorial in the Danish

Figure 1.2. Melting snow to make tea while the dogs rest. Dr. Dyerberg is on the right.

Medical Society's weekly journal pointed out the unusual pattern of heart disease among the population of Inuits or Eskimos who were Danish citizens living in the part of Denmark named Greenland. The major part of the world's Inuits were at that time Danish citizens. It was the editor's opinion that Danish medical doctors had an obligation to research the medical peculiarities that existed— before it was too late, meaning before Westernization of the Inuit society took over—when comparing the populations in the two parts of the Danish kingdom: Denmark and Greenland.

I was at that time resident physician at Dr. Bang's laboratory at the city hospital of Aalborg. Dr. Bang had been conducting intensive research in lipid-related risk factors for coronary heart disease. He had found, as had other lipid researchers, that a high blood level of cholesterol was a major risk factor for that, and the culprit was a high intake of fat in our diets. Dr. Bang had visited Greenland in the 1950s when a measles epidemic struck the then-virgin population, causing severe illnesses. He suggested that we should respond to the journal's call to action and revisit Greenland to perform plasma lipid analyses on Eskimos living in their original way.

The surprising information in the editorial was namely that the Eskimos, in spite of a high fat content in their traditional diet, did *not* have a high coronary heart disease incidence—quite the contrary, a very *low* incidence! Could that be due to the composition of the marine fats they lived on? Upon reading this editorial, Dr. Bang said to me, "I guess no one else is going to be collecting samples from Inuits who hunt and fish any time soon, so let's take samples and publish the results so at least people will know what the blood parameters were in the 1970s." I agreed that the world was changing fast and the window of opportunity was short. So we dropped everything else we were doing and devoted ourselves to obtaining these samples while there was still time.

Obviously, these were solid scientific reasons to examine the Eskimos' blood lipids to see if these, in spite of high fat consumption, were as favorable as the low coronary heart disease incidence indicated!

Important factors in coronary heart disease development are in the blood proteins that transport fats and cholesterol. Fats and cholesterol are not soluble in blood, which is largely water, and must be transported in proteins called *lipoproteins*. Lipoproteins are "friendly" to both water and fats. They carry the fats inside their structures whose outsides are compatible with water and blood. At that time I had nearly finished my doctoral thesis based on a new method for measuring the various lipoproteins in blood. I had developed an agarose-based electrophoresis method that would enable us to determine not only the blood lipids in Eskimos, but also the blood lipoproteins—if only we could get up there and sample their blood. We had to do the analyses on the spot, as lipoproteins in the blood are unstable and could not be shipped to Denmark for analysis.

A lot of clerical work had to be done before undertaking the expedition. It included applications to the ministry of Greenland, the health authorities, and other government officials and not least to apply for money for such an expedition—monies to buy and ship equipment, both personal and analytical, for a month-long stay for three people in the wilderness. We finally managed to collect $5,000 for our expedition to collect blood from Eskimo hunters and fishermen and their families.

On Our Way

We were now on our way to Igdlorssuit, but we were basing our operations out of a small town on the coast of Baffin's Bay called Umanak because it had both electricity and a hospital. Incidentally, as it turns out, *umanak* means "heart" in Inuit. Perhaps you may recognize *igloo* in the name Igdlorssuit, which translates to "the big houses."

The trip was cumbersome. We had to fly from Copenhagen to the American air base in Sondrestrom, Greenland. From there, a helicopter took us to the city of Egedesminde. We then boarded a cargo boat that also carried a few passengers and delivered us some days later farther up the Greenland west coast.

We were well received at the small twenty-bed hospital in Umanak and were kindly invited to join the doctor on his trips to the small settlements in the Uummannaq district, where about 100 people lived at each one. The families depended on the hunter-fisherman's ability to provide the family with food. As I've mentioned, their traditional diet was based on seal and fatty fish, and now and then a small whale. Western food items were sparse, mostly sugar and biscuits.

By necessity, the Eskimo diet is different from diets of those living in warmer climates. The snow- and ice-covered Arctic with its long periods of darkness is not conducive to growing plants, so isolated villages depend mostly on fishing and whatever else they can find hunting for food. The classical food pyramid for U.S. citizens has fats, oils, and sweets in the smallest section with the recommendation to use them sparingly. Figure 1.3 depicts how the Eskimo food pyramid might look to an outsider. Needless to say, it's quite different than the U.S. food pyramid!

I lived on Eskimo provisions on many occasions and grew quickly fond of raw seal liver with a helping of fresh seal blubber and a meal of dried seal meat. The food we ate was identical to the Eskimo protein- and fat-rich diet, with very little carbohydrate. We also ate the seal intestines, after turning them inside out and washing them by dragging them after the boat. The sled dogs also liked these meals, and I had to be on guard to defend my meals from them. I carried fairly large sticks or stones for this purpose. Towns here usually had a ratio of ten dogs for every person, but the dogs are not pets.

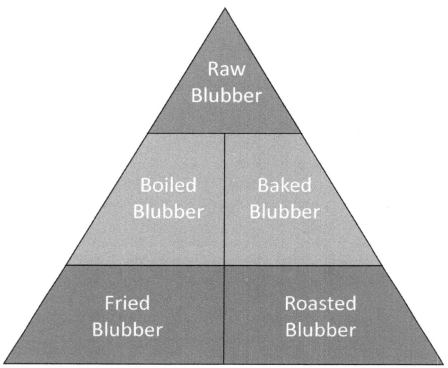

Raw
Blubber

Boiled
Blubber

Baked
Blubber

Fried
Blubber

Roasted
Blubber

On reflection today, my experience in Greenland was very pleasant. It

Figure 1.3. How the Eskimo food pyramid might seem to outsiders.

was more than the thrill of the science; it was the enjoyment of the people and the land as well. In our five Greenland expeditions, the scientific results of which made a turning point in human nutrition by discovering the role of omega-3 fatty acids' essentiality in heart health and their unique physiological effects, we in heart health enjoyed the *experience* of going out there in the wilderness!

Being a young doctor in my thirties, science was of course my priority on the tours, *but* I shall not underestimate the value of having had the opportunity to experience what many are not given. On some expeditions we chose to go in April or in August to take advantage of the long Arctic days. However, the almost endless daylight was not conducive to sleeping, and thus we had the opportunity to explore and play. We were able to go sailing, kayaking, and dogsledding for days. We ate raw seal and whale, and slept on floors in schools and churches in sleeping bags and in houses in remote places. I even shot birds and caught fish myself (I never shot a seal but have been on hunting tours with Eskimo hunters who did). Certainly the science was and is of a very high value for me, but the personal experiences I had during those scientific endeavors I shall never forget.

Collecting Blood Samples

Now, back to our scientific detective work: We managed at our first expedition in 1970 to collect blood from 130 Eskimos, males and females. The blood lipid and lipoprotein analyses that we did at the laboratory in Umanak showed uniformly a low content of the triglyceride-containing very low-density lipoprotein (VLDL). VLDL contains the highest amount of triglycerides, the main form that fats are carried in the blood and a known risk factor for heart disease. This was the first indication of what we know today, namely, the strong triglyceride-lowering effect of the omega-3 fatty acids: EPA (eicosapentaenoic acid) and DHA (docosahexaenoic acid). However, we would later find that EPA and DHA have even more important effects to reduce the risk of heart disease.

After returning to Denmark we finished analyzing the blood samples and in April 1971 published the article "Plasma Lipid and Lipoprotein Pattern in Greenlandic West-Coast Eskimos" in the reputed medical journal the *Lancet* (Bang, 1971). Even though the word *omega-3* was never mentioned in this seminal article, the editor notes, "These early observations were crucial in formulating a hypothesis to account for the low incidence in coronary heart disease in a population consuming a high-fat, high-cholesterol diet." The study has since been classified as a "nutrition classic."

Nonetheless, we had to conclude that even though the Eskimos had favorable blood fat levels, they were *not* low enough to explain why these remote-living Eskimos had only about one-tenth the incidence of heart disease compared with Danes and Americans. Thus we had to search for additional explanations. What could they be?

Testing for Clues

The first thing we did was to get an old gas chromatograph working again that Dr. Bang had in his lab. For readers not familiar with gas chromatography, it was an early analytical instrument that was used to separate and quantify individual compounds of a mixture. Since we weren't looking for anything special, our goal was to determine whatever we could about the Eskimo blood fat profiles with our 130 samples and then compare the fatty acid composition with that of typical Danes. The research was hard work, but we felt it was our duty to analyze and learn as much as we could before the Eskimos' diet and traditional way of life were altered.

As I said, we were just testing for everything we knew about, but we did notice a couple of extra peaks in the chromatogram analysis of the blood samples from the Eskimos—peaks that we had never noticed before. We didn't know what these mystery compounds indicated, but it was reasonable to believe that they were fatty acids. We didn't know if one or both of them were related to the mystery. So I sought help in the interpretation of our results from Dr. Ralph Holman at the Hormel Institute in Minnesota, who was the leading fatty acid analyst of the time.

Judging from the position of the peaks, Dr. Holman postulated that we had found omega-3 fatty acids in the blood, quite possibly EPA and DHA. I still remember repeating these two strange names—eicosapentaenoic acid and docosahexaenoic acid—just to learn them. At that time no notice was given to these fatty acids in either human medicine or nutrition. (We'll describe these missing wellness factors in more detail in Chapter 3.)

Eventually, after years of research and several more expeditions, we detailed our findings "Fatty Acid Composition of Plasma Lipids in Greenland Eskimos" in the *American Journal of Clinical Nutrition* (Dyerberg, 1975). We concluded that "If dietary differences are the main reasons for the differences in coronary heart disease incidence in Eskimos, the results from this study point toward *qualitative* differences in respect of fatty acid composition of the food." But I'm getting ahead of myself.

Back to Greenland

It would take years in the interim to discover where EPA and DHA came from, if they were related to heart disease, and if so, how. We consequently were to find these two fatty acids in the Eskimo food! The focus of our next two expeditions to Greenland in 1972 and 1976 was to collect and analyze the Eskimo food and to see if we could find the explanation in the food for their favorable blood lipid levels—despite their high fat diet. No one had done that before.

We did that in both summer- and wintertimes (1972 and 1976, respectively) with a special focus on EPA. By that time, we had found a very high content of EPA (and DHA) in Eskimo blood. We were still working with the analysis to be published in 1975, but we had seen these fatty acids in many samples in 1972. I wrote—very foresighted as it turned out to be—in 1972 in the first food-collecting expedition diary: "This fatty acid (EPA) can only come from the food, as our bodies cannot make it. Even if any connection between a component that unique and lowering of coronary disease risk at present is purely speculative and completely unfounded, it opens up for very wide nutritional perspectives and justifies fully a detailed analysis of the original Eskimo food."

What we did at these two expeditions to Igdlorssuit was to sample the food the Eskimos were living on, by asking the volunteers to use the double-portion food-collection technique. We supplied them with plastic bags and asked them to put exactly the same sort and amount of food in the plastic bag as they ate at every meal during the day. We then the next morning bought the bag after many friendly price negotiations. What is the price of a fresh seal eye, considered a special delicacy? I have had it, and it tastes good, but it is a bit difficult to chew. Every one of our volunteers cooperated perfectly; even the hunters, on hunting trips for days, brought back their plastic sacks with raw meat and seal liver.

We used a generator to give us electricity to run a meat grinder and a blender. We then weighed a sample of a day's homogenized provision and froze it. We did not have a freezer, but used an ice and salt mix in an isolated box we had built. Such a salt-ice mix can have a temperature of zero Fahrenheit, and there was plenty of ice to sample! The rest of the minced provisions were given to the huskies, of which approximately 900 ran freely around on the island, when they were not working as sled dogs. Greenland huskies are *not* pets, and even if you feed them, you should never try to caress them. They are tough, and never come into the houses. A heavy stick is a good thing to have in your hand when close to them.

The results from both expeditions were strikingly similar to the fatty acid analysis of the 130 blood samples published in the *American Journal of Clinical Nutrition*. At that time we had found the key to "unlocking the Eskimos' nutritional treasure"—our special fatty acids EPA and DHA that had unexpected and hitherto unknown biological effects. This brought us to the end of our first three expeditions. As we would discover over the next two expeditions and in subsequent years, each has separate functions, and they are not merely two of the same. Table 1.1 chronicles our expeditions to Greenland and the principal purpose of each expedition. We could now shift our focus from what these mystery compounds were to discovering just what each has to do with human health.

Onward.

TABLE 1.1. RESEARCH SUMMARY OF SCIENTIFIC EXPEDITIONS TO GREENLAND		
DATE OF EXPEDITION	PRINCIPAL LOCATION	PRINCIPAL PURPOSE OF EXPEDITION
August–September 1970	Umanak (Uummannaq) district Greenland	To examine the blood lipids and lipoproteins in traditionally living Eskimos
August 1972	Igdlorssuit settlement in the Umanak district	To collect and examine Eskimo food, during summer period
April–May 1976	Igdlorssuit settlement in the Umanak district	To collect and examine Eskimo food, during winter period
July–August 1978	Igdlorssuit settlement in the Umanak district	To examine cutaneous bleeding-time and platelet aggregation in traditionally living Eskimos
July–August 1982	Umanak (Uummannaq) district Greenland	To examine blood pressure in traditionally living Eskimos

"Eicosa What? Docosa What?"

At this point in our story, we have established that a difference between the blood of Greenland Eskimos and their Danish co-citizens in Denmark is that the Eskimos' blood contained eicosapentaenoic acid and docosahexaenoic acid in high amounts. You may be thinking, "Eicosa what? Dicosa what?" If the terms *eicosapentaenoic* and *docosahexaenoic* (pronounced *eye-co-sa-pen-tah-i-no-ic* and *do-co-sa-hex-a-e-no-ic*) sound Greek to you, be assured that they do at first to many scientists. Don't be put off by their long names; you don't have to pronounce them or use them. Most people, including scientists, merely call them by their acronyms: EPA and DHA.

Even though these compounds are called *acids,* they are not harsh chemicals normally associated with the word *acid*. In fact, these acids are weaker than common acids found in foods such as fruit acids or acetic acid in vinegar. They are fatty acids, which don't react or attack normal body compounds, but only react with the help of enzymes with certain compounds like glycerol to form fat compounds.

Fats perform many vital roles in our bodies. In fact, some readers may be surprised to learn that fats are essential to our health (especially to heart and brain health!) and protect us against many diseases. It is often written that there are "good fats" and "bad fats." However, there are really no bad natural fats, only bad quantities of fat intake. (Man-made trans fats, which are produced by a manufacturing process called *hydrogenation,* are one exception; more on these fats later.) Even the often-maligned saturated fats associated with animal fats have their roles in maintaining proper membrane functions and transporting fat-soluble vitamins. But this too is a concept for later discussion.

BASIC FATTY ACID ANATOMY

Fatty acids are the basic units or building blocks of fats. All life is based on the biochemistry of compounds containing the element carbon. Carbon is the second-most plentiful element by weight (behind oxygen) in the body, typically at 18 percent, and the third most plentiful element in terms of the number of atoms (9.5 percent). We will gradually work our way to explaining why EPA and DHA are called omega-3, long-chain polyunsaturated fatty acids (or omega-3 LC-PUFAs, a term we'll be using frequently, so keep it in mind), but for right now you don't have to be concerned with this concept. The only thing that is really important to know about EPA and DHA now is that their chemical structures are unique and they have two important functions because of these unique structures.

We require both of these specific nutrients for optimal health because of their unique vital functions. Even though EPA and DHA are related structurally and usually occur together, they are distinct compounds having unique functions. EPA cannot replace DHA, nor can DHA replace EPA; even though the body can convert small quantities of each into the other, that amount is not adequate for good health. Unfortunately, EPA and DHA levels in modern diets are inadequate and are disappearing rapidly. Other nutrients, even fatty acids of the same omega-3 family other than EPA and DHA, cannot perform the vital functions of EPA and DHA. As we will discuss later, this is because of their chemical structures as very long, very unsaturated molecules. The vital functions of EPA and DHA will be described in the following chapter, but for now let's interrupt Dr. Dyerberg's recounting of his exciting scientific detective story to discuss the basic biochemistry of fatty acids, and specifically the importance of EPA and DHA's chemical structures.

One note: Our mission in writing this book is to help you live better longer, not to teach biochemistry to readers less interested in "why" and more interested in "how" EPA and DHA do what they do. We feel it's important that everyone learn how to optimize their health and reduce their risk of many serious diseases and disorders presented in the later chapters, so we don't want readers to think this book is getting too technical and have some give up before they get to the important parts. So if the following discussion seems to be more than you want to know, or if you'd rather keep on reading about Dr. Dyerberg's adventure and discoveries, just skip ahead to the next chapter. No one is looking and there will be no quiz. You can always come back here for clarifications if needed.

We would be remiss, however, if we didn't present the following background and correct a few misconceptions. Understanding the basic terminology and the definitions helps explain the uniqueness of these omega-3 fats and their special health benefits. This brief background may answer some of the questions going through your mind. Give it a shot. We promise that this will be the only chapter reviewing very basic biochemistry rather than results. We also promise that you will be interested in the results given in the later chapters!

CHEMICAL STRUCTURE

Chemicals, including fatty acids, are assigned descriptive names by scientists based on their chemical structures. However, because EPA and DHA have become of interest only relatively recently, their scientific names were widely adopted and their trivial names—timnodonic acid and cervonic acid—are rarely used. The scientific names eicosapentaenoic acid and docosahexaenoic acid spell out to chemists that these compounds have twenty and twenty-two carbon atoms, respectively, linked together with an acid group on one end. The affixes *eicosa* and *docosa* are from the Greek words for "twenty" and "twenty-two"; the suffix *oic* means each has a carboxylic acid group. (We will leave the *penta* and *hexa* portions of our explanation for later.) Let's take this step by step.

Short-, Medium-, and Long-Chain Fatty Acids

A fatty acid molecule is a chain of carbon atoms with hydrogen and oxygen attached. It has two terminals (ends) and a middle chain. The length of the carbon chain and the number and type of bonds between some of the carbon atoms determine the type of fatty acid it forms. Scientists like to think of molecules as not really having beginnings and ends, just terminals (ends). Would you describe a person as having a beginning and an end? Some people would consider one's head the beginning and their feet the end. Other people would do the opposite. In nature, molecules don't know which terminal (end) is a "beginning" and which is an "end." They rotate at high speeds, and it is their structures that determine how they interact with other molecules.

Fatty acids vary in the number of carbon atoms they have. Normally, a fatty acid has between three and twenty-two carbon atoms in the mid-chain portion of its molecule, although there can be more. One carbon atom is located in each of the terminal groups. Figure 2.1 shows the basic structural backbone of a fatty acid. The methyl terminal (left), which is sometimes called the *omega* end, consists of a carbon atom with three hydrogen atoms. The end of the fatty acid farthest from the methyl group is the acid group. This carboxyl terminal (right), which is sometimes called the *alpha* end, consists of a carbon atom with two oxygen atoms and a hydrogen atom.

Fatty acids found in foods come in different chain lengths, ranging in total carbon atoms from three carbons (a short-chain fatty acid) to between eight and fourteen carbons (a medium-chain fatty acid) to twenty-two or more carbons (a long-chain fatty acid). Most fatty acids made in the body are shorter in chain length.

Carbon atoms are linked in a zigzag fashion in the molecule due to

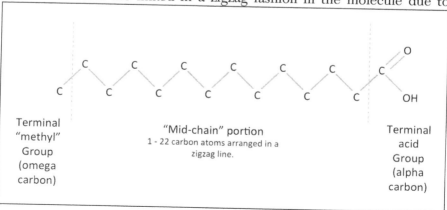

Figure 2.1. Carbon atom "backbone" arrangement in a saturated fatty acid.

forces of the electrons orbiting their nuclei, so they look like zigzagging strings. It may be easier to understand the structural differences among various fatty acids if you think of the carbon atoms strung together like a string of pearls. Neither "chain" nor "string" is a perfect analogy, but the carbon atoms behave more as if they are strung together on a zig-zagging wire than chains links in a chain. This will be apparent later, but for now let's stick with the common analogy of chain in order to follow the long-chain polyunsaturated fatty acid concept.

In nature, carbon atoms are neither chained together nor strung together, but are held in place by electromagnetic forces that are generated when atoms share certain electron orbitals. The bonds are properties of the electron orbits as they share two atoms; in the case of the carbon chains of fatty acids, two carbon atoms. These forces are called *bonds*, and the important differences between single bonds and double bonds will be discussed shortly. Right now what is important to know is that fatty acids have structures that vary in length, according to the number of carbon atoms they contain and the types and numbers of bonds between those carbons, and that these factors determine their functions in the body. The health benefits that we will describe in later chapters are due solely to the actions of the long-chain polyunsaturated fatty acids, EPA and DHA. Short- and medium-chain fatty acids do not have the same health benefits as long-chain fatty acids.

An Ideal Structure for Storage, Transport, and Use

Fatty acids are the basic units or building blocks of dietary fats and oils. EPA and DHA, like all fatty acids, are weak acids. Remember from earlier in the chapter that organic acids within the body are usually weak acids because they don't readily release the hydrogen atom in the acid group like strong acids such as hydrochloric acid do. However, this weak ionization is favorable for forming fat compounds called *triglycerides.*

Fats typically exist as three molecules of fatty acids combined with a glycerol molecule to form—you guessed it—a triglyceride. Its shape is favorable for storing fatty acids compactly in the body and for transporting them easily in the blood. Normally, the fatty acids in a triglyceride are three different fatty acids and not three of the same fatty acid. Often there is at least one unsaturated fatty acid in the triglyceride, but there can be virtually any combination of saturated and unsaturated fats. When fatty acids are not attached to other molecules, they are known as "free" fatty acids.

Fats and oils found in food are present mostly in this triglyceride storage or transport form, and not as unattached free fatty acids. And like fats in the body, fats in food normally consist of various triglycerides composed of various fatty acids. Thus, fat in foods are mixtures of fatty acids in triglyceride form. Each food contains different amounts of various triglycerides, which help give each food a different taste and feel.

The metabolic processes within the body use these fatty acids when needed to make other fat-related compounds such as *phospholipids*—the principal components of every cell membrane—and *eicosanoids*—powerful hormonelike substances synthesized from the twenty-carbon fatty acids in these phospholipids. We will discuss phospholipids and eicosanoids in detail in later chapters when we explain how EPA and DHA function to bring about their myriad of health benefits.

We should mention that fats and oils are essentially the same types of chemical compounds, differing only in their physical forms at ambient temperature in their native source. Chemists simply call them both *lipids*. As a general rule, if a lipid is solid at ambient temperature, it is what most people call a *fat;* if the lipid is liquid at ambient temperature, it is what most people call an oil. A fat's physical form—solid or liquid—depends mostly on the size of the molecule and the amount of saturation and unsaturation.

SATURATED AND UNSATURATED FATTY ACIDS

If you are not a chemist, we congratulate you for surviving and learning all this new nomenclature about the basics of fatty acids. There is just one more important concept to understand about fatty acids: saturated vs. unsaturated types. This will help in understanding how the long-chain polyunsaturated fatty acids EPA and DHA do what they do, and lead to an understanding of the importance of the term *omega-3*. In this discussion we will set straight a few myths and misunderstandings about fats.

Whether a fat is saturated or unsaturated depends on the structure of the fatty acid and the amount of hydrogen present in it. When all the carbon atoms in a fatty acid molecule are paired up with hydrogen atoms, the fat is "saturated," or completely filled. If a fatty acid is not fully saturated, it is said to be "unsaturated." Hydrogen is the most plentiful element in the body—and in the universe—in terms of the number of atoms of the element; it typically makes up 63 percent of all atoms in the body. When compounds are composed of carbon and hydrogen, they are called hydrocarbons. In the body, the three elements carbon, hydrogen, and oxygen account for 93 percent by weight and 98.4 percent of all the atoms. Since the body typically contains 75 percent (65 to 90 percent range) water (consisting of hydrogen and oxygen), this is not surprising.

Fatty acids are mostly made up of carbon and hydrogen, with the exception being the "acid" terminal of the molecule, which contains two oxygen atoms in addition to carbon and hydrogen.

Saturated Fatty Acids

The carbon atoms in a saturated fatty acid are fully loaded with hydrogen and appear in an inflexible straight line, although in a zigzag arrangement. The electrons around the carbon atoms in saturated fatty acids are relatively stable, with fewer intermolecular forces and actions taking place. Also, some scientists believe that the zigzag pattern of the carbon chains of fatty acids allows them to pack closer together much like nested boxes and this gives them a firmer structure. They have a similar effect in cell membranes.

Figure 2.2 (on the following page) illustrates how hydrogen atoms are arranged on the carbon chain backbone of a saturated fatty acid.

Skeletal molecular structures, which are simplified, less-cluttered diagrams of fatty acids that do not show every carbon and hydrogen atom, are easier to understand and will be used most frequently here, after one or two more basic explanations. See Figure 2.3 (also on the following page) for an example of the "skeletal" representation of a saturated fatty acid.

Fats that are made up of triglycerides having mostly saturated fatty acids tend to have higher melting points and are usually solid at ambient temperature. If they are totally saturated, they are waxy and difficult to

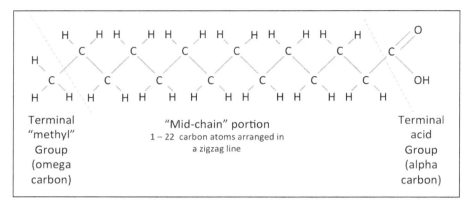

Figure 2.2. Adding the hydrogen atoms (represented by the letter "H") to a saturated fatty acid.

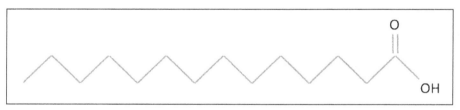

Figure 2.3. Skeletal representation of a saturated fatty acid in which the "C" for carbon atoms is eliminated as well as the "H" for the hydrogen atoms attached to the chain carbons; the "O" for oxygen and the one "H" for hydrogen in the acid group are retained.

digest. Totally saturated oils are rare in nature. Natural fats, animal or plant, are normally mixtures of both saturated and unsaturated fatty acids.

A common misconception is that animal fats are saturated fats, and, conversely, that saturated fats are animal fats. Well, some are and some aren't. Fish are not plants, yet they are rich in unsaturated fatty acids. Coconut oil, from the fruit of the coconut plant, is 85 percent saturated fat. As lipid expert Dr. Mary Enig points out in her book *Know Your Fats* (2000), "The practice of calling animal fats 'saturated' is not only misleading, it is just plain wrong. For example, beef fat is 54 percent unsaturated; lard is 60 percent unsaturated; and chicken fat is about 70 percent unsaturated. This makes these animal fats less than half saturated. Therefore, they really should be called unsaturated fats." The inset below includes more surprising fat findings.

BODY FAT AND OLIVE OIL RICH IN MONOUNSATURATED FATTY ACIDS

Because fats and oils are mixtures of fatty acids, animal fats and plant oils often contain some of the same fatty acids. As an example, the fatty acid oleic acid is found in many fats and oils, both of plant origin and animal origin. Oleic acid is exactly the same chemical compound regardless if it comes from animals or plants. This monounsaturated fatty acid is often considered the essence of the Mediterranean diet, as olive oil is 78 percent oleic acid. However, the fat in eggs is 50 percent oleic acid; beef tallow is 48 percent oleic acid, lard is 44 percent, and cow's milk is 33 percent. It is not surprising that oleic acid is the most abundant fatty acid in adipose tissue, or body fat. It can be said that humans are an example of an animal rich in monounsaturated fatty acid, oleic acid!

Plants and animals can produce both saturated and unsaturated fatty acids. There's also good reason why the human body makes both—they are needed for optimal health. Saturated fats provide structure for cell membranes and are a critical source of energy in important organs such as the heart. Plants and animals contain enzymes called *desaturases* that can remove certain hydrogen atoms in saturated fatty acids to produce unsaturated fatty acids. Humans, however, are limited in their ability to convert saturated fatty acids into the unsaturated form. EPA and DHA are two essential unsaturated fatty acids that humans cannot produce and thus must obtain from their diet. We will discuss these dietary essential fatty acids in detail in Chapter 5, but right now let's focus on unsaturated fatty acids.

Unsaturated Fatty Acids

Unsaturated fatty acids include mono- and polyunsaturated fatty acids. The carbon atoms in these fatty acids are not completely paired with hydrogen atoms. They have less than the maximum number of hydrogen atoms than their carbon backbones can hold. The number of unsaturated carbons in a fatty acid determines its shape and function. When hydrogen atoms are removed from a saturated fatty acid (making it an unsaturated fatty acid), the electrons orbiting the carbon atoms assume a different orbital. This change results in different electromagnetic forces and influences the positions of the carbon atoms. A kink or bend, known as a double bond, is formed in the zigzag configuration as two carbon atoms now share an additional electron. Keep in mind that the term *double bond* refers to the force holding atoms together in a molecule, a property not of the elements, but their orbiting electrons.

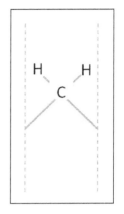

Let's look back for a moment at saturated fatty acids to better understand double bonds. Each mid-chain carbon atom in a saturated fatty acid is paired (or shares) electrons with two neighboring hydrogen atoms as in Figure 2.4, as well as two neighboring carbon atoms (not shown).

When hydrogen atoms that were formerly attached to neighboring carbon atoms are removed, the two carbon atoms now have to share an electron with each other. The result is a double bond. Figure 2.5 illustrates the formation of a double bond in an unsaturated fatty acid.

Figure 2.4. Mid-chain carbon atoms in a saturated fat have two hydrogen atoms attached.

The greater the degree of unsaturation (that is, the more double bonds), the greater the likelihood that the fatty acid will be liquid at ambient temperature. Fewer hydrogen atoms are attached to the carbons to "stiffen" the molecule. They have a similar effect on cell membranes.

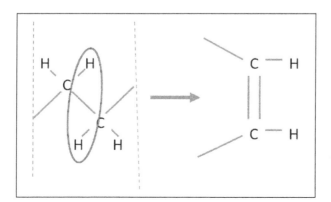

Figure 2.5. Formation of a double bond. After two hydrogen atoms are removed from the adjacent carbon atoms, the atoms rearrange themselves so that the hydrogen atoms are on the same side of the double bond.

Monounsaturated Fatty Acids

A fatty acid that contains only one double bond is called a *monounsat-urated* fatty acid, or MUFA. The best-known example of a monounsat-urated fatty acid is oleic acid, the principal fatty acid in olive oil. The skeletal structural representation for the MUFA, oleic acid, is shown in Figure 2.6.

Polyunsaturated Fatty Acids

A fatty acid that has more than one double bond is called a *polyunsat-urated* fatty acid, or PUFA. As the number of dou-

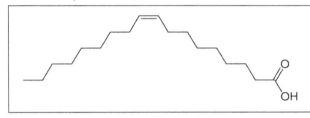

Figure 2.6.
The skeletal structure of the monounsaturated fatty acid oleic acid.

ble bonds increases, the molecule bends, occupying more space. Most vegetable and fish oils are rich in PUFAs.

PUFAs, in turn, are further classified by numbering the location of the first double bond counted from the methyl terminal (omega end). Double bonds prevent molecules from freely rotating about their own axis. The normal electron arrangement in these double carbon bonds is a *cis* bond. Cis is Latin for "on the same side." For decades, it was thought that cis formation forces molecules to have kinks or bends. Modern instruments that can more exactly view chemical structures are modifying this earlier observation. The molecule naturally readjusts its structure to have the lowest energy level, but it appears that certain low-energy changes in conformation can take place in certain carbon atoms in PUFAs, and PUFAs can exist in several conformation states (structures).

At the double bonds, however, the lowest energy conformations are accomplished by repositioning the involved hydrogen atoms on the same sides of the double bond. Cis double bonds not only cause the fatty acid molecule to bend, but they also stiffen the bend. The result is a more space-filling molecule that requires less energy for the body to form into eicosanoids, the class of hormonelike molecules mentioned earlier that are converted from the fatty acids found in cell membranes. The more cis double bonds in a fatty acid molecule, the more pronounced the bent shape can become. Studies of long-chain polyunsaturated fatty acids (LC-PUFAs) suggest that they have add additional movement and flexibility in the carbon atoms between the double bonds (Stillwell, 2003). Four, five, and six double-bond fatty acids can have circular or ring shapes.

An abnormal rearrangement of the electrons results in a *trans* double bond. (Remember the hazardous trans fats we warned you about in the beginning of the chapter?) Trans double bonds, or trans fats, are formed artificially during a man-made process called *hydrogenation.* Examples can also be found in nature in ruminants (grazing farm animals such as sheep and cattle). Man-made trans fats cause alterations to numerous physiological functions of cell membranes and are harmful to health, as we will discuss in Chapter 5. Figure 2.7 illustrates cis and trans isomers (configurations or variants) of a double bond.

The positions of the double bonds in PUFAs are more important than their number, but both factors are important, as you'll now see.

THE OMEGA FAMILY OF FATTY ACIDS

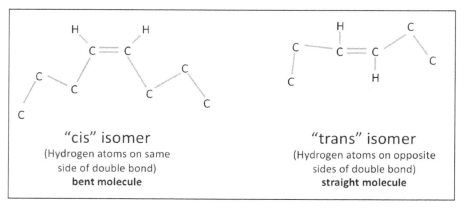

"cis" isomer
(Hydrogen atoms on same
side of double bond)
bent molecule

"trans" isomer
(Hydrogen atoms on opposite
sides of double bond)
straight molecule

Figure 2.7. Cis and trans double bonds. In a cis double bond (left), the hydrogen atoms are on the same side of the double bond, causing the molecule to bend; in a trans double bond (right), the hydrogen atoms are on the opposite sides of the double bond, causing the molecule to straighten.

Congratulations! You've covered a lot of chemistry to get here, but finally, you're at the heart of the matter. What's important now are the positions or locations of the double bonds in the fatty acids—especially the first double bond from the methyl terminal (the end opposite the terminal with the acid group). There are strong health benefits from the fatty acids that have their first double bond as close to the end as possible—at the third carbon from the end.

Omega is the last letter in the Greek alphabet, so the carbon atom in the methyl terminal can be considered the last carbon in the fatty acid; that's why it is called the *omega* carbon. We will always spell out omega, but often the Greek letter itself (ω) or even the letter *n* (meaning "end") is used. Counting from the omega carbon, the third carbon from this end is called the *omega-3* carbon (omega minus three). If there is a double bond at this carbon, the fatty acid is called an *omega-3 fatty acid.* The omega-3 family of fatty acids contains short-, medium- and long-chain varieties, but the only omega-3 fatty acids that produce the special health benefits described in this book are the LC-PUFAs, EPA and DHA.

Earlier in the chapter, we said that EPA and DHA had two important functions because of their unique structures that are critical to health and the prevention of many common diseases and disorders.

Their first major function is as basic compounds in cell membranes where they are easily stored. Think of them as building blocks for all cell membranes that make up the body's 60 trillion cells. They are responsible for the fluidity in the cell membrane that makes possible the movement of biochemical and messenger compounds about the membrane that have important cell-regulating functions throughout the body and the flow of nutrients and harmful cellular waste into and out from the cell. DHA particularly impacts the fluidity of cell membranes in the brain, where it supports proper development and functioning of the brain and nervous system. Membrane walls rich in EPA and DHA help prevent cellular damage that can eventually result in disease.

The second function unique to EPA and DHA is that they can be converted in cell membranes into a class of powerful hormonelike messenger compounds called *eicosanoids* and *docosanoids* that affect virtually every system in the body. Certain eicosanoids—prostaglandins, leukotrienes, and thromboxanes—provide the unique health benefits of EPA such as keeping blood flowing freely and regulating pain and inflammation. Regulating inflammation is critical, since it's now thought to be a causative factor in many serious chronic disease. Certain docosanoids—protectins, resolvins, maresins, and others—provide health benefits unique to DHA that we describe later when we get back to Dr. Dyerberg's Greenland Eskimo adventure.

Other important unsaturated fatty acids include members of the omega-6 and omega-9 families. As you guessed, their first double bonds are located on the omega-6 carbons and omega-9 carbons, respectively.

Why is the location of the first double bond so important? Figure 2.8 illustrates how different each type is because of this difference in distance from the omega carbon.

Omega-3 Fatty Acids

The major omega-3 fatty acids are alpha-linolenic acid (ALA), eicosapentaenoic (EPA), and docosahexaenoic acid (DHA). The omega-3 family is headed by ALA, the shortest-chain member from which longer-chain members can be derived. Omega-3 fatty acids are found in some vegetable oils, fish, and seafood. ALA is particularly abundant in flaxseed,

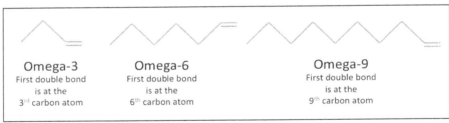

Omega-3
First double bond
is at the
3rd carbon atom

Omega-6
First double bond
is at the
6th carbon atom

Omega-9
First double bond
is at the
9th carbon atom

Figure 2.8. The nutritionally important omega families.

canola, soy, perilla, and walnut oils. EPA and DHA are found predominately in marine creatures, including fish, krill, squid, octopus, as well as from marine algae.

Humans have a biochemical pathway in the liver, gut, and brain that can convert some of the omega-3 fatty acid ALA into EPA and DHA. This is accomplished via enzymes that can elongate and desaturate the precursor fatty acids. The rate of conversion of ALA to EPA is below 5 percent, and ALA to DHA is negligible (Plourde, 2007). ALA is considered dietary essential, whereas EPA and DHA are considered semi-essential. (The essentiality of fats will be discussed in Chapter 5.) These low rates of conversion are insufficient to achieve tissue levels of EPA and DHA that are protective against many diseases and disorders.

We are not implying that short-chain or medium-chain omega-3 fatty acids are not important. We need to increase the quantity of all the omega-3s in our diets to better utilize the enzymes that can convert short-chain omega-3s into EPA and DHA. Therefore, more omega-3 of all types in the diet is beneficial, but we emphasize that the diet should contain at least 1 gram (1,000 milligrams) of EPA and DHA (combined), regardless of how much of the other omega-3s are present.

Figure 2.9 shows the structure that the omega-3 fatty acid ALA has the greatest probability of forming at any given time. The atoms in a PUFA such as ALA are in motion and can move about in and out of several different conformations (arrangements). Notice that the three double bonds bend the molecule considerably so that it occupies more space in a cell membrane, which makes it more fluid and pliable.

Omega-6 Fatty Acids

The primary fatty acid in the omega-6 family is linoleic acid (LA), an eighteen-carbon polyunsaturated fatty acid having two double bonds. Like the omega-3 ALA, LA is considered a dietary essential fatty acid. It is the precursor to arachidonic acid (AA). AA is a twenty-carbon polyunsaturated omega-6 fatty acid having

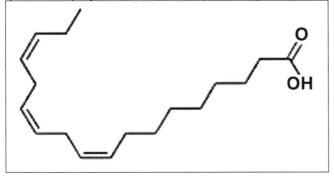

Figure 2.9.
The most favorable conformation structure for the omega-3 alpha-linolenic acid.

four double bonds. It is often confused with the saturated twenty-carbon fatty acid arachidic acid found in peanut oil and corn oil. LA is found in seed oils like corn, safflower, soy, and rapeseed.

Compare the structure of omega-6 LA in Figure 2.10 with that of omega-3 ALA in Figure 2.9. Both have eighteen carbons, but the number of double bonds and location of the first double bond differ. Note the difference in molecular shape caused by the number of double bonds. LA is a straighter, more rigid molecule that occupies less space.

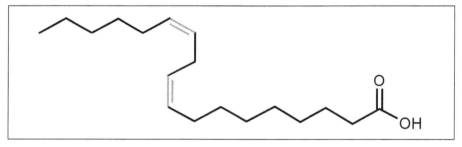

Figure 2.10. The most favorable conformation structure for the omega-6 fatty acid linoleic acid.

Omega-9 Fatty Acids

The omega-9 monounsaturated fatty acid oleic acid is also an important dietary fatty acid. Its structure was shown in Figure 2.6, and if you remember, it's almost a linear molecule. This is because it has only one double bond.

UNIQUE AMONG FATTY ACIDS

Now we can finish our explanation of the nomenclature for EPA (eicos-apentaenoic acid) and DHA (docosahexaenoic acid). As we alluded to earlier and will provide evidence for throughout this book, nothing else—no other compound—not even other omega-3 fatty acids can do what EPA and DHA can do! It's not just that EPA and DHA are *longer* molecules, it's that they have *more* double bonds and are *bent* into shapes that allow eicosanoids and docosanoids to be quickly and easily formed.

EPA

We started by explaining that *eicosa* was Greek for twenty and *oic* designated "acid." Now we add *penta*, which means "five." Thus, the name eicosapentaenoic acid tells us that it is a fatty acid containing twenty carbon atoms and five double bonds. The structure for EPA is shown in Figure 2.11 (below). Notice that the molecule almost forms a horseshoe shape. This facilitates its conversion into various

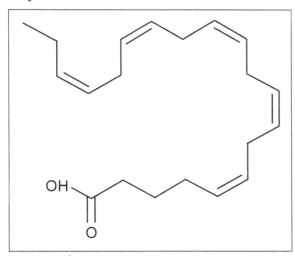

Figure 2.11.
One of the most favorable conformation structures for the LC-PUFA EPA. This horseshoe shape makes it easy for EPA
to form eicosanoids.

eicosanoids.

DHA

Similarly, docosahexaenoic acid is a unique twenty-two-carbon fatty acid having six double bonds. *Docosa* is Greek for "twenty-two," *oic* means "acid," and *hexa* means "six." One of the most favorable conformations of its molecular structure is shown in Figure 2.12. The six double bonds in a DHA molecule not only help facilitate its conversion into various docosanoids but also keep the molecule in motion, which can be said to be responsible for our ability to think and see.

Well, now you know much more about EPA

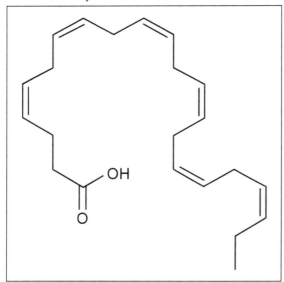

Figure 2.12.
The DHA structure is far from linear. Its six double bonds allow sufficient molecular motion to help keep cell membranes fluid.

and DHA than Dr. Dyerberg did when he discovered them in the blood of Eskimos. Remember, they may be commonplace terms now, but they were not known to have a function in the body before Dr. Dyerberg uncovered them and their clinical importance in heart disease in the 1970s in Eskimos. Only a few scientists who specialized in the chemistry of food fats paid much attention to them. The molecular structures of EPA and DHA give them unique properties that account for their far-reaching health benefits. Although they are similar in chemical structure, they do not have identical functions, so we must obtain both from the diet for optimal health.

What did their presence in the Eskimo blood mean? Could they be responsible for protecting the Eskimos against heart disease? Were they real clues or just incidental artifacts? Let's get back to the detective work of Dr. Dyerberg and his colleagues.

3

The Missing Links

Now that we better understand what EPA and DHA are and how they function, we can get back to Dr. Dyerberg's detective story and see how these omega-3 long-chain polyunsaturated fatty acids (LC-PUFAs) are involved in protecting us from heart disease. Let's return to Dr. Dyerberg's accounts of how he and his colleagues solved the scientific mystery.

CLUE BY CLUE

By 1976 we had made three expeditions to Greenland to discover how these Eskimos could live in such a remote place on a fat-rich diet and still have remarkably low rates of heart disease. The journeys added up in years and miles. We had to travel from Denmark to Greenland to Denmark to the United States to Denmark and back to Greenland gathering clues and consulting with experts in other fields to put all of the pieces together. We had found EPA and DHA in all classes of blood fats: free fatty acids, triglycerides, cholesterols, and phospholipids. The question now was, what is the meaning of these findings? Are they just incidental artifacts, or do they serve some physiological purpose? Are EPA and DHA also in the blood of typical Danes like myself, and are just somehow overlooked? We were at a loss to explain the anomaly. So we decided to look further for them—this time in the blood of typical Danes.

We used our blood lipid findings collected from 130 Greenland Eskimos during our first expedition in 1970, and compared the composition to thirty-one Danes and thirty-two Greenland Eskimos living in Denmark. We did find EPA and DHA there too, but at very much lower levels. They had been missed in earlier comparisons because the amounts were too low to be noticed, unlike the relatively large amounts we found in the Eskimo blood, which were so large they attracted our attention.

A Chance Finding

Despite these new findings, we still had no clue as to how EPA and/or DHA could be relevant to heart disease. By chance, we had also noticed that the Eskimos' blood samples were lower in another fatty acid called *arachidonic acid* (AA). At that time, scientific discoveries were coming out of Sweden and England showing that blood clotting, among many other things, was regulated by compounds called *prostaglandins* formed from AA.

Prostaglandins are now recognized as members of the larger eicosanoid family of fatty acids. In the 1930s, a compound originating in the prostate gland and isolated in seminal fluid was discovered to stimulate contraction of the uterus. But it wasn't until about 1972 that Drs. Bergström and Samuelsson (in Sweden) and Dr. Vane and his group (in England) discovered that compounds with similar chemical structures affected platelet aggregation and, in turn, platelet stickiness and blood clotting. Platelets are small, disk-shaped bodies in the blood that promote clotting, but when clumped in hardened arteries, they can cause heart attacks and strokes. Bergström, Samuelsson, and Vance were awarded the Nobel Prize in Physiology or Medicine in 1982 for their research.

Prostaglandins are synthesized in the body from AA and, as we later learned, also from EPA. AA is a polyunsaturated fatty acid found in some animal fats, including fish, and is made in the body from the omega-6 fatty acid, linoleic acid (LA). AA can form leukotrienes and members of the E2 series of the prostanoid family of eicosanoids, which include prostaglandins, prostacyclins, thromboxanes (Enig, 2000); all compounds that increase inflammation and blood platelet activation, which in turn increase the tendency for blood to clot. (Both actions will be explained in Chapters 4 and 8.) AA has a chain length of twenty-carbon atoms, the same number as EPA; but it has only four double bonds, whereas

EPA has five. The important difference, though, is that EPA has its first double bond in the omega-3 position and AA has its first double bond in the omega-6 position.

We then hypothesized that the shift in the Eskimos' blood from AA to EPA could "tune" their blood clotting into a less active state by changing the prostaglandin formation to compounds generated from EPA. That would in turn diminish the risk for clots in their arteries and consequently their risk of heart attacks. The role of blood clotting in heart disease made a lot of sense to us. Most heart attacks are due to blood clots, formed on a hardening (plaque) in the heart's arteries. Keeping the blood slippery and free from clotting will reduce the probability of having the common heart attack.

In our lab, we investigated whether EPA could give rise to the formation of prostaglandins, which have an effect on blood clotting. This, we found, fit with our hypothesis of an "anti-clotting" effect of EPA on blood. Our search for more answers was to take us back to the Arctic to study the Eskimos' blood and diets once again.

The Missing Links

It was during this fourth expedition to northern Greenland in 1978 that we confirmed that EPA affected the clotting time of the Eskimos' blood. We studied this by measuring the Eskimos' bleeding tendency and found they actually had a longer cutaneous bleeding time than the Danes. That it took longer for their blood to clot suggested that the blood clots did not form in their coronary arteries as easily or as quickly. In 1979, again in the *Lancet*, we reported our results in a paper entitled "Haemostatic Function and Platelet Polyunsaturated Fatty Acids in Eskimos." This paper also became a nutrition classic.

Despite our findings we still had yet to discover where EPA and DHA came from. Back then not much was known about EPA and DHA. Human beings don't produce many long-chain omega-3 fatty acids in their bodies, and polyunsaturated fatty acids were associated with plant foods, not animals. What we found was that although fish and seals don't make EPA and DHA themselves, they consume and concentrate these omega-3 fatty acids from the foods they eat. EPA and DHA are synthesized in the sea's biosphere by phytoplankton (marine algae). The EPA and DHA made in the algae are then passed up the food chain to bigger and bigger organisms and finally to the fatty cold-water fish or, as for the Eskimos, seals that live on fish into humans. Fish living in cold water need to store more body fat for survival and thus become good reservoirs of fatty acids. Good examples of such fish include mackerel, cod, salmon, herring, sardines, and tuna.

You may remember from Chapter 1 that when we returned to Greenland in 1976, we collected food from the Eskimos using the cumbersome double-portion technique, homogenized the food, and froze it to be transported for analysis in Denmark. We had found from our analyses that the Eskimos on average ate approximately 14 grams of omega-3 LC-PUFAs, mostly EPA and DHA per day!

SHARING THE MISSING TREASURE

The next question then became: Could the positive effects on the heart and arteries of EPA and DHA omega-3 fatty acids from fish and fish oils in the Eskimos be transferred to our society by supplementing our diet with EPA and DHA from fish oils? That's a question that today, after forty years of research and after undertaking approximately 22,000 studies of volunteers and patients with heart diseases, can be answered with an unambiguous "yes."

A 2009 survey of the preventable causes of deaths in the United States concludes that 84,000 deaths per year are attributable to low-dietary omega-3 fatty acid intake (Danaei, 2009)! Furthermore, we have today obtained extensive insights into how this beneficial effect is brought about. The studies have found that EPA and DHA omega-3 LC-PUFAs from fish oils have several positive effects that work in combination, thereby lowering the risk of heart attacks, stroke, and other diseases. The same is true for patients already suffering from heart disease.

To best understand the benefits of these omega-3 LC-PUFAs, let's take a brief look at the roles of prostaglandins and the other eicosanoids that EPA produces, along with the docosanoids that DHA produces.

4

Eicosanoids and Docosanoids Fine-Tune Body Chemistry

A t the time that Dr. Dyerberg's group observed that a shift in Eskimos' blood from omega-6 arachidonic acid (AA)–rich fatty acids to omega-3 EPA- and DHA-rich fatty acids tuned their blood into a less-active clotting state by changing the prostaglandin formation, research on prostaglandins and their larger family of eicosanoids was just in its initial state. By diminishing the risk of clots in the Eskimos' arteries, these omega-3 long-chain polyunsaturated fats (LC-PUFAs) diminished their risk of heart attacks.

A heart attack is caused by the formation of a thrombus, or a blood clot, in one of the coronary arteries that supplies the heart muscle with blood. The clot is formed in the artery where an atherosclerotic plaque has formed within the artery wall and forced the wall inward, which narrows the opening (lumen) of the artery. When treating patients with a propensity toward blood clotting, doctors prescribe anti-coagulant drugs such as warfarin (Coumadin) and heparin to reduce the tendency for clots. As found in Eskimos, omega-3 fatty acids regulate the blood's own clotting system such that the clotting tendency is lowered; this is primarily due to the effect of EPA (although studies in 2011 suggest that DHA may possibly have a similar role by another mechanism now under study). EPA is converted to a group of eicsoanoids that tune the clotting system toward a lower level of activity than when eicosanoids are only formed from AA, which heighten the activity. It is important to note that the shift is rather modest, and does not give rise to concern regarding bleeding risk (see "It's Safe to Go with the Flow" on page 36).

IT'S SAFE TO GO WITH THE FLOW

In Eskimos who eat more than 10 grams of omega-3 fatty acids a day, a tendency to experience nosebleeds has been observed. The most frequently recommended dosage of EPA and DHA is 1 gram daily for general nutritional purposes. With special medical conditions as arthritis and high triglycerides, physicians often recommend up to 4 grams daily. An increased tendency to bleed is not observed at these levels. People taking prescribed anti-coagulants (such as warfarin or heparin) should check with their physician regarding EPA/DHA supplementation.

At first this ability to prevent or promote blood clotting was thought to be the sole role of eicosanoids. Since these initial findings, research has found that eicosanoids play an even more powerful role in preventing or promoting inflammation, which can make the difference between being healthy and having non-germ disorders such as heart disease and cancer. And while it may seem that eicosanoids derived from EPA have health-supporting positive effects and those derived from AA are harmful and can cause the opposite effect, that's simply not the case. Both omega-3 eicosanoids and omega-6 eicosanoids perform important functions in the body. So let's briefly discuss them. No need for more biochemistry—just a couple of quick definitions will help readers understand the relationship between EPA- and AA-derived eicosanoids, and the many body functions that each performs. The relationship is readily apparent once you are given a couple of facts.

OMEGA-3 AND OMEGA-6 EICOSANOIDS

Let's pick up our explanation of eicosanoids where we left off in Chapter 2. Eicosanoids are a group of hormonelike compounds that are formed in the cell membranes from twenty-carbon omega-3 and omega-6 polyunsaturated fatty acids. Eicosanoids are like hormones in that they control many basic functions. The important difference between them, however, is that hormones are produced in a specific gland (like the thyroid or pituitary) and then travel primarily through the bloodstream to regulate body functions such as breathing and heart rate. As that takes time, hormones tend to have a long life span before they are degraded. In contrast, eicosanoids are produced on the spot in every cell membrane (not in one specific gland) and then are released. They act locally and nearly instantly (usually in response to trauma) to regulate functions at the cellular level. As such, eicosanoids have a very short life span; they do their job and are immediately destroyed by neighboring enzymes or oxidizing compounds. Unlike hormones, the body cannot store eicosanoids but must manufacture them when needed from the omega-3 and omega-6 fatty acids stored in phospholipids in cell membranes.

There are two main categories of eicosanoids: prostanoids and leukotrienes, along with several minor categories. Prostanoids include prostaglandins, prostacyclins, and thromboxanes. Within each category of eicosanoid, there are several types of prostaglandins, several types of leukotrienes, and so on. To differentiate them from one another, they are further grouped into various series. Each of these eicosanoid series is referred to by a letter, followed by the number of the series it belongs to: for example, prostaglandin A1 or leukotriene A2. Eicosanoids in the same series tend to have similar effects.

Omega-3 and omega-6 LC-PUFAs each produce a series of eicosanoids that are characterized as the 3-series or 6-series. Table 4.1 lists a few of the important biological processes that each series performs.

TABLE 4.1. DIFFERENT FORMS AND FUNCTIONS OF EICOSANOIDS

EICOSANOIDS DERIVED FROM OMEGA-3 EPA	EICOSANOIDS DERIVED FROM OMEGA-6 AA
Reduce blood clotting	Increase blood clotting
Dilate blood vessels (decrease high blood pressure)	Constrict blood vessels (increase blood pressure)
Cause weak inflammatory response	Cause strong inflammatory response
Dilate air passages	Constrict air passages
Reduce pain	Promote pain
Enhance the immune system	Depress the immune system
Improve brain function	Decrease brain function
Decrease swelling	Increase swelling
Decrease inflammation (additional anti-inflammatory action comes from DHA-derived docosanoids)	No such actions

Eicosanoids derived from omega-3 EPA and those from omega-6 AA have balancing effects on one another. For example, the 3-series prostaglandins and 5-series leukotrienes from EPA are favorable to a healthy cardiovascular system and can lessen inflammation. AA produces eicosanoids of the 4-series leukotrienes and the 2-series prostanoids that *in excess* can be harmful to the cardiovascular system by stimulating inflammation. It's not simply a matter of "good" and "bad" eicosanoids, but a matter of balance. Similarly, eicosanoids in differing series tend to balance one another's actions. For example, thromboxanes such as thromboxane A2 promote platelet aggregation (stickiness), whereas prostacyclin I2 inhibits platelet aggregation in the blood. The body needs enough thromboxane A2 to ensure healthy clotting, yet it must have enough prostacyclin I2 to protect against unhealthy clotting, which can lead to heart attacks and strokes. It's this constant tug-o-war between the eicosanoids that allows the body to be fine-tuned for optimal health. We don't want an excess of either, but rather depend on a balance of the two.

Eicosanoids and Diet

Eicosanoids (*eicosa* means "twenty" in Greek) are made from the twenty-carbon omega-3 and omega-6 PUFAs. Because the body is unable to produce either omega-3 or omega-6 PUFAs, they must be obtained through the diet. The body has a limited amount of special enzymes that can lengthen fatty acid chain length and increase the number of double bonds (thereby increasing its unsaturation). Thus, to a very limited extent some LC-PUFAs can be made in the body from short- or medium-chain PUFAs, but more LC-PUFAs have to come from the diet to optimally meet the body's needs. Since the amount of these special enzymes is limited, the omega-3 and omega-6 PUFAs compete with each other to use these special enzymes to form LC-PUFAs. In addition, the formation of eicosanoids from LC-PUFAs requires other enzymes, and once again, the LC-PUFAs, AA and EPA, must compete for these enzymes.

A diet of either more or less omega-3 or omega-6 therefore plays a crucial role in affecting the balance essential for regulating eicosanoid production. A diet rich in the omega-6 fatty acids from meat (the chief dietary source of AA), grains, and vegetable-seed oils (the chief source of linoleic acid)—abundant in the Westernized diet—encourages the production of pro-inflammatory eicosanoids. In contrast, a diet rich in omega-3 fatty acids from marine creatures, including fish, krill, squid, octopus, as well as from marine algae, or EPA/DHA supplements from these sources encourages the production of anti-inflammatory eicosanoids. As we shall see next, excessive production of pro-inflammatory eicosanoids can lead not only to heart disease but also to many other serious diseases and disorders.

HELP FROM THE DOCOSANOIDS

The twenty-two-carbon omega-3 DHA produces a family of hormonelike compounds called *docosanoids*. These include resolvins, protectins, and maresins, which are extremely potent compounds. Like the eicosanoids, docosanoids have important anti-inflammatory properties. They are also thought to function as neuroprotectins in the brain and throughout the entire central nervous system where DHA is abundant. Resolvins of the D-series (DHA-derived) are produced from DHA. Protectins are also formed by these pathways. Resolvins are mediators that can powerfully clear inflammation by removing excess neutrophils and macrophages (white blood cells that initiate inflammation) from inflammatory sites. Interestingly, EPA also gives rise to production of E-series resolvins with twenty-carbon atoms in their molecule, and with similar effects as those generated from DHA. This is in contrast to the situation for AA, from which no such components are synthesized.

Both EPA and DHA reduce platelet aggregation, but in slightly different ways (see "Partners in Health" on page 40). A study in 2011 showed that a single dose of EPA or DHA can decrease the activity of platelets by 20 percent. This study, conducted at the University of Newcastle in New South Wales, Australia, found that a single dose of EPA-rich oil significantly inhibits platelet activity and subsequently reduces platelet aggregation, while supplementation with DHA-rich oils reduces platelet aggregation independent of platelet activity. The total amount of EPA and DHA was 1,000 milligrams (mg) or 1 gram in each group, with the EPA-rich group receiving a single dose of 0.833 mg of EPA plus 0.167 mg DHA, while the DHA-rich group received a single dose of 0.167 mg EPA plus 0.833 mg DHA (Phang, 2011).

PARTNERS IN HEALTH

EPA and DHA are not merely replacements for each other. DHA is not just another EPA. They are related structurally and are usually found together, but they have different and distinct biological functions. EPA cannot directly substitute for DHA, nor can DHA directly replace EPA. The body can convert a small amount of one to the other, but still the biochemistry of EPA, which has a twenty-carbon chain with five double bonds, is different than that of DHA, which has a twenty-two-carbon chain with six double bonds. An important difference is that EPA can form twenty-carbon compounds called *eicosanoids*, while DHA can form twenty-two-carbon compounds called *docosanoids*. Eicosanoids and docosanoids are distinct families of compounds. A docosanoid is not just another eicosanoid. EPA and DHA, as well as their derivatives, are both important and are needed by the body. They both have become "the missing wellness factors." An important distinction is that prostaglandins, one of the families within the larger eicosanoid family, have a major, direct influence on blood clotting. Thus, EPA directly affects blood-clotting tendencies via mechanisms reducing platelet aggregation, whereas DHA affects blood-clotting tendencies via mechanisms independent of platelet aggregation.

PRO-INFLAMMATORY AND ANTI-INFLAMMATORY EICOSANOIDS

It was surprising to many scientists that inflammation was found to be a causative factor in many diseases—not just a result of having these diseases. This may still be a new concept to many readers, so let's discuss how inflammation works and why this process exists. Knowing a little about the inflammatory process will help you understand how EPA and DHA reduce inflammation and the risk of inflammation-related diseases.

Inflammation and Chronic Disease

Inflammation is a protective attempt by the body to heal an injury and to help remove the injurious agent whether it is of physical, chemical, or infectious origin. The word *inflammation* stems from the Latin word meaning "to set on fire," and that is because the inflammatory process generates heat. Doctors use the Latin shortlist *calor, dolor, rubor,* and *tumor* (meaning "heat," "pain," "redness," and "swelling") to describe an inflammatory process. This complex process is vital to survival, as it fights the inflammatory agents.

Inflammation can be classified as either acute or chronic. Acute inflammation is the classical initial localized response of the body to harmful agents. The body's inflammatory system treats the injury or infectious agent or irritant immediately and returns the body to health. Prolonged inflammation, known as chronic inflammation, is the opposite of acute. In chronic inflammation, the body's inflammatory response is unable to heal the injury or eradicate the unresolved trigger, so it is perpetually activated. This leads to a progressive shift in the type of cells present at the site of inflammation and is characterized by simultaneous destruction and healing. Instead of staying localized, the inflammatory response spreads. This type of chronic low-grade inflammation is often referred to as "silent inflammation" or as a "silent fire within" because it often goes undetected in the early stages. We prefer to use the term "uncontrolled inflammation" to indicate its systemic, perpetual nature. The destructive nature of low-grade, persistent inflammation can lead to many diseases. Uncontrolled inflammation can result as an aging immune system loses its ability to function properly.

Once the only chronic diseases considered inflammatory illnesses were asthma (inflamed airways) and "-itis" diseases such as arthritis (inflamed joints), allergic rhinitis (hay fever), colitis (inflamed bowel), dermatitis (inflamed skin), sinusitis (inflamed sinuses), and gingivitis (inflamed gums). *Itis* is merely the suffix for inflammation of an organ. Since then, our understanding of inflammation has grown considerably as has the list of conditions associated with chronic inflammation. For example, heart disease is now considered to result from uncontrolled low-grade inflammation in the coronary arteries; many cancers are considered to result from chronic uncontrolled inflammation in the cells; and Alzheimer's disease is thought to be the consequence of inflammation in the brain that leads to the buildup of a protein called *amyloid*. In fact, a growing body of research now suggests that low-grade inflammation is one of the key components in many chronic diseases, either as a cause or promoter of the disease process.

People with chronic inflammatory disease often endure a great deal of suffering. Because their inflammation cannot be fully controlled, many turn to medications such as non-steroidal anti-inflammatory drugs (NSAIDs) and even steroids to relieve the pain, fatigue, digestive problems, and other symptoms caused by the inflammation. But all of them have their own side effects. Some people also find that their symptoms and struggles are dismissed by others, who cannot fully understand the debilitation of living with a chronic inflammatory disease.

Inflammation can be measured by a simple blood test for C-reactive protein (CRP), a substance that is both a promoter and a marker of low-grade inflammation. CRP is part of the family of cytokines, cell-communication molecules, that tells cells to release all sorts of pro-inflammatory substances. The presence of CRP in blood is a sign of inflammation because it is normally not present in appreciable amounts in the blood of health people. But while the CRP test measures the level of inflammation in the body, it cannot yet indicate where the inflammation is coming from. (For readers who want to learn more about how inflammation plays a fundamental role in disease, we recommend *The Inflammation Syndrome* by Jack Challem.)

Potent Natural Anti-Inflammatories

The first protective effect of EPA that was identified was that it prevented blood clotting that causes heart attacks. However, soon other benefits from EPA and its ability to form additional and more diverse eicosanoids became apparent. The natural anti-inflammatory effect of this omega-3 LC-PUFA was first noticed when examining the chemotactic potency (meaning the ability to "call on" leukocytes to participate in an inflammatory process) of leukotrienes formed from EPA compared to leukotrienes formed from AA. Leukotrienes derived from AA exhibit ten- to thirtyfold greater pro-inflammatory response than leukotrienes derived from EPA (Lee, 1984). In addition to the ecosanoids, it is now believed that docosanoids are needed to bring inflammation under control.

Current anti-inflammatory therapies are directed toward the inhibition of specific enzymes and/or the antagonism of specific receptors. The widely used cyclooxygenase (COX) inhibitors are examples of this approach. COX inhibitors, the common analgesics known as NSAIDS, interfere with the chemical enzyme cyclooxygenase, which in turn blocks the production of pro-inflammatory chemical mediators that cause pain and inflammation. Recent research has uncovered new mechanisms that terminate or resolve the acute inflammatory response locally. These are active processes and the resolution, that was once considered a passive process, is actually an active process at the tissue level. Thus, rather than targeting inhibition, the focus of current research is on addressing the potential use of agonists (substances that bind to cell receptors and trigger a response) to stimulate key endogenous (inside the body) regulatory points within the control of mechanisms that naturally resolve inflammation. In other words, this new approach focuses on stimulating chemical pathways within the regulatory mechanism that keeps inflammation both able to be activated and yet be held in check.

The identification of new families of lipid mediators generated from omega-3 LC-PUFAs, and *not* from omega-6 LC-PUFAs, helped further this understanding (Serhan, 2002, 2010, 2011). Compounds such as E-series resolvins, D-series resolvins, protectins/neuroprotectins, and, most recently, maresins are both pro-resolving and anti-inflammatory and appear to play a physiological role in terminating inflammation. These lipid mediators are synthesized in the body from EPA and DHA exclusively (see "Meet the New Families" for more on the special properties of these pro-resolving and anti-inflammatory substances). There are no known counterparts synthesized from AA.

MEET THE NEW FAMILIES

Omega-3 LC-PUFAs, in contrast to omega-6 LC-PUFAs, are precursors to new families of lipid mediators that are both pro-resolving and anti-inflammatory and appear to play a physiological role in terminating inflammation, including E-series resolvins, D-series resolvins, protectins/neuroprotectins, and, most recently, maresins. Each family appears to have a specific role in targeting inflammation.

- Resolvins were coined with this term because they are generated during the resolution phase of inflammation. Experimental evidence indicates that resolvins reduce cellular inflammation by inhibiting the production and transportation of inflammatory cells and chemicals to the sites of inflammation.

- Another chemical family was coined protectins, because in animals, specific members of this family control the duration and magnitude of inflammation. They were originally found in brain tissue, and were consequently called neuroprotectins. They have since been found to be synthesized in many organs aside from the brain.

- The term *maresin* is coined from macrophage mediators involved in resolving inflammation (maresin). They were found to possess potent anti-inflammatory and pro-resolving properties similar to resolvin E1.

While these substances are just being discovered, the beneficial effects of eicosanoids and docosanoids are well known to people with arthritis who experience pain relief due to attenuation of the inflammatory process when taking fish oil supplements. Given the potent pro-inflammatory actions of leukotrienes in disease, our daily intake of EPA and DHA may attenuate the development of cardiovascular diseases. As will be discussed in Chapter 8, Heart Disease, inflammation within the artery walls can interact with and oxidize low-density lipoprotein (LDL) particles of a certain size and contribute to plaque formation commonly called *cholesterol deposits*. The LDL itself does not play a primary or initiating role in this process. In the same way, omega-3 fatty acids can attenuate the inflammatory process in the vessel walls and thereby the progression of the atherosclerotic process.

Evidence of this is that people with high omega-3 intake have lower CRP levels in the blood than those with a low omega-3 intake. Remember, CRP rises during inflammatory processes in the body. People with elevated levels of CRP are at an increased risk for ischemic heart diseases (IHDs), the most common cause of death in most Western countries. IHD is the medical term for reduced blood flow to the heart, usually due to a clot-related obstruction of blood flow. This is true even for apparently healthy men and women who have normal blood cholesterol levels. By lowering the inflammatory activity in the body, supplementation with EPA and DHA adds an extra protective facet to the broad spectrum of beneficial effects of omega-3 LC-PUFAs on ischemic heart diseases. In 2009, a study led by Dr. M. Garg of the University of New Castle in

New South Wales, Australia, found that increased blood levels of EPA and DHA were associated with reduced levels of CRP (Micallef, 2009).

These findings are consistent with a 2011 clinical study led by Dr. J. Virtanen at the University of Eastern Finland in which he concluded, "Serum omega-3 PUFAs and especially the long-chain ω-3 [omega-3] PUFA concentration, a marker of fish or fish oil consumption, were inversely associated with serum CRP." The study examined blood omega-3 PUFA levels and blood CRP levels in 1,395 healthy Finnish men, ages forty-two to sixty, using data from the prospective, population-based Kuopio Ischemic Heart Disease Risk Factor Study. High EPA/DHA blood levels were associated with low CRP levels. The study found an especially strong inverse relationship with blood EPA level and blood CRP level (Reinders, 2011). In a study a year later, researchers found that "Fish oil [EPA] has been associated with anti-inflammatory gene expression, for example, with decreased expression of nuclear factor-κB (NF-κB)" (Magee, 2012). In other words, EPA suppresses the production of NF-κB, a substance in cells that is responsible for regulating the expression of genes involved in inflammation—an important new finding that may help further explain the powerful actions of EPA.

As Dr. Dyerberg's group uncovered the benefits of EPA and DHA in the Eskimo's blood and other scientists discovered more actions of the eicosanoids, a new picture was unfolding that captured the interests of even more scientists.

5

Essential Fats

ats are essential to life. Some fats are dietary essential, meaning they are nutrients that are absolutely essential for good health, but they cannot be produced by the body and, therefore, must be obtained from a food source or supplement. Some fats are semi-essential under certain conditions such as pregnancy and a child's first few months of life; and some, in particular, industrial-produced trans fats, are harmful and should be avoided. At one time, fats were considered merely unessential sources of calories. Now, we understand that fats are important components of every cell and that the many compounds made from these fats are involved in controlling thousands of functions.

So why are some fats beneficial and some trans fats are not? Where and how do we come by them? Let's find out.

ESSENTIAL FATTY ACIDS

The concept of the essentiality of certain dietary fatty acids (usually just called essential fatty acids, or EFAs) was developed decades ago. The first evidence of the essentialness of certain fats in the diet was observed by Dr. George Oswald Burr. In 1924 Burr, then a young doctoral graduate, went to the University of California, Berkeley, to help Dr. Herbert McLean Evans and Dr. Katherine Scott Bishop with their research on vitamin E. Two years earlier, Evans and Bishop had discovered what they called the "anti-sterility factor" in the fat portion of laboratory rat diets. At first they called it vitamin X but soon changed it to vitamin E.

Evans and Bishop were having trouble reproducing their results and Burr thought that his expertise in fat-free diets would be useful. Burr helped concentrate, identify, and determine the physiology of vitamin E in several joint papers with Evans in the late 1920s.

However, the research indicated to Burr that another missing nutritional factor in dietary fat was causing the infertility. In the meantime, Burr and the group's overseer of their laboratory rat colony, Dr. Mildred Lawson, were married in 1925. Their emerging research with fat-free diets led them to postulate that fats contained an essential dietary factor.

Their thesis—that certain dietary fats might be essential nutrients—was not well received within the scientific community; not even by their colleague Dr. Evans. New ideas in science are often met with resistance, especially from scientists who may feel they have intellectual "territory" to protect. Besides it was "well known" that the only function of fats was to transport fat-soluble vitamins and to store calories that could later be used as a source of energy. After all, it had previously been proven that animals could readily make fats from carbohydrates. Although the Burrs' finding had surprised even them, they saw the evidence pointing to an essential dietary factor in dietary fat that could not be ignored.

Essential Fats for Growth and Reproduction

At the time, scientists reasoned that because the body could make its own fats from carbohydrates, it would have no need to take fats from the diet. What the recently married couple had astutely noted, and what other scientists had missed, was that the fats created in the body were hard and more saturated, whereas the fats stored in the animals' bodies were softer and more unsaturated and tended to proportionally reflect the amount of unsaturated fats they consumed in their diet. We now know that fats made in the body are saturated and monounsaturated fats, which are harder and less fluid than polyunsaturated fats (PUFAs). Pliable and soft, unsaturated fats are ideal for forming cell membranes and for making eicosanoids and docosanoids.

When the lab rats were fed diets that lacked PUFAs, they became unhealthy. When PUFAs were added back into the animals' diets, they became healthy again. Other scientists pooh-poohed the Burrs' concept of a fat being essential, and instead suggested that another vitaminlike factor was missing from the animals' fat-free diet. Soon the Burrs moved from their Berkeley laboratory to the University of Minnesota.

In 1927 the preliminary evidence on the essentiality of vitamin E was published jointly by Dr. Evans and Dr. Burr in the *Journal of Biological Chemistry*. For the next two years, George and Mildred Burr attempted to disseminate the concept of EFAs to the scientific community on their own. They continued to be ridiculed by their colleagues. They maintained that linoleic acid (LA)—an eighteen-carbon omega-6 fatty acid, which cannot be made in the body of animals—was involved.

In 1929 the Burrs published their results in the same journal and identified this fatty acid as an essential nutrient for rats. They reported that a fat-free diet impaired the growth and reproduction of laboratory animals. Moreover, the animals developed other symptoms. They formed scaly skin and consumed excessive quantities of water; they lost weight, their tails became necrotic and dropped off, and their kidneys degenerated, which led to blood in their urine. These symptoms were eliminated when LA was added to the animals' fat-free diet. However, to increase the chances of having their research accepted, they positioned the missing factor as a vitamin rather than as a dietary PUFA. They called this factor *vitamin F.*

The concept was accepted slowly but steadily. When researchers tried to apply the animal findings to humans they could not do so at first, because they did not realize that it took months for humans to deplete their reserves of EFAs.

As George Burr recounted, "When William Anderson wrote his review of recent advances [in the *Yale Journal of Biology and Medicine* in 1932], he put it something like this: 'The Burrs offer for serious consideration the view that certain fatty acids are essential constituents of animal diets.' Do you detect a note of skepticism? But we soon had many supporters. You now have at hand the hundreds of papers that have been written on the amounts needed, the relative values of various acids, the need by other animals, ranging from insects to Homo sapiens. The review I wrote for the *Federation Proceedings* in 1942 was pretty good up to that time."

Twenty-Five Years Later

Studying fat metabolism in animals on a fat-free diet is one thing, but inducing an EFA deficiency in humans is another. The human body retains fats—especially PUFAs—for extremely long periods of time. Eventually, in the 1960s, the concept of EFAs surreptitiously reemerged when intravenous feeding using total parental nutrition (TPN) began. The nutrient mixture used to feed patients unable to eat was fat free. These TPN solutions led to the same symptoms in patients such as scaly skin and excessive thirst that had been observed in fat-deficient laboratory animals.

Interestingly, George Burr happened to be the faculty advisor for Ralph Holman (introduced in Chapter 1), who was the expert Dr. Dyerberg sought out to help identify the unknown peaks he found in the blood of the Eskimos. Our story is almost coming full circle.

In time, Dr. Holman assumed the Burrs' line of research. He demonstrated with his own studies that feeding animals the essential LA increased the amount of arachidonic acid (AA) in their bodies. Also, feeding animals the essential alpha-linolenic acid (ALA) slightly increased the amount of EPA, and to even a lesser extent, DHA.

The concept of essential fatty acids is odd in a way in that, except for having a function in the water barrier of the skin due to incorporation of LA into phospholipids in the skin of EFA-deficient rats, no direct use for LA has ever been found. Studies have shown that LA is essential by being incorporated into two skin fats (acylglucosylceramide and acylceramide). The results of animal experiments indicate that re-establishment of a low water loss through the skin was associated with incorporation of LA into the two lipids in the skin. No direct use for ALA has been found at this writing. The primary function of these two EFAs in the body is to produce the long-chain PUFAs (LC-PUFAs), EPA, DHA, and AA, which are needed to form cell membranes and to make eicosanoids from EPA and docosanoids from DHA.

Semi-Essential Fatty Acids

As far as body function is concerned, EPA, DHA, and AA are "function-ally essential." To scientists, however, at this writing (but we trust this will change), only ALA and LA are considered "dietary essential." This is because some EPA, DHA, and AA can be made from them in the body. The enzyme reactions that convert ALA into EPA and DHA fail to satisfy the full need for EPA and DHA by the body. Therefore, EPA and DHA must also be supplied in the diet to avoid the risk of deficiency. Because of this, they can be said to be "conditionally essential" or "semi-essential."

The synthesis of LC-PUFAs from their dietary precursors (ALA and LA) is slow and limited. The body has a limited amount of elongase and desaturase, enzymes that are required to lengthen and add additional double bonds to the shorter-chain PUFAs. Moreover, the same enzymes are required to make both omega-3 and omega-6 PUFAs and the two fatty acid families compete for them. As a result, there are often inadequate amounts of these enzymes to meet the body's optimal needs. Therefore, the diet needs to supply optimal amounts not only of the so-called essential PUFAs, but also of their long-chain derivatives.

Because of this competition between ALA and LA for the same limited quantities of these enzymes, if the body has to process an overabundance of one omega family, it can cause a deficiency of the other omega family. In the typical Western diet, which contains very high amounts of omega-6 LA, the result is that little EPA and nearly no DHA is produced from omega-3 ALA.

It was Dr. Holman who found that ALA and LA need the same set of enzymes to produce the LC-PUFAs needed for producing eicosanoids and docosanoids. In doing this research, Holman found it more convenient to describe these fatty acids based on the methyl terminal as being either omega-3 or omega-6 fatty acids, rather than the awkward scientific nomenclature based on the acid terminal (all-cis-9,12,15-octadecatrienoic acid and all-cis 9,12-octadecadienoic acid, respectively). Normally, chemists prefer to put emphasis on the acid end of a molecule, but now, they find it more useful to emphasize the tail omega end of the fatty acid molecule. This makes our understanding so much easier. The first description of this omega terminology appeared in Holman's 1964 article in the *Journal of Lipid Research.*

It wasn't until about 1970 that medical authorities realized that EFAs were critical to the retina (more on this in Chapter 15). Now, we recognize that EFAs in sufficient quantity are essential not only for reproduction and normal growth and development, but also for good health.

Dietary Sources of Omega-3 and Omega-6 EFAs

The primary source of omega-3 fatty acids in the diet is ALA. The most concentrated sources of ALA are found in flaxseed, canola, soy, perilla, and walnut oils. Many commonly eaten dark leafy greens are also adequate sources of this fatty acid. Cold-water fish (such as salmon, sardines, mackerel, anchovies, and other fatty species) as well as krill, squid, octopus, and marine algae and their oils are considered the most important dietary sources of omega-3 because they contain the most concentrated amounts of the longer-chain EPA and DHA.

Few Americans reach the recommended levels of intake of the omega-3 fatty acids. Some estimates suggest Americans get only a single-digit percentage of the recommended levels of intake for omega-3 fatty acids. There are no definitive guidelines concerning optimal intakes of EFAs. However, in 2002 the Institute of Medicine at the National Academy of Sciences, a non-profit organization that provides unbiased, evidence-based information and advice concerning health and science policy to policymakers, issued Adequate Intake (AI) levels for ALA, the initial building block of all omega-3 fatty acids found in the body. For male teenagers and adult men, 1.6 grams per day were recommended; for female teenagers and adult women, the recommended amount was 1.1 grams per day.

The primary source of omega-6 fatty acids in the diet is LA. In the body, LA is converted to AA, which is not technically considered essential because, in perfect circumstances, our bodies are able to make adequate amounts of AA out of LA. Like ALA, LA cannot be made by the body and must be supplied by the diet. LA is found in seed oils like corn, safflower, soy, and rapeseed—oils abundant in processed and packaged food, and thus plentiful in the Western diet. AA is found in animal fats, especially pork, and to a lesser extent, also in fish oils.

The recommended daily intake for omega-6 fatty acid is about 2–3 percent of daily calories. Most of us consume far more than that due to the disproportionate amount of omega-6 fats in the current Western diet. Nearly 7 percent of total calories in the typical fat-rich American diet come from PUFAs.

ALA CONVERSION TO EPA AND DHA

At the time Dr. Dyerberg's team made their original observations of the Eskimos, the essentiality of fatty acids was thought to apply only to LA, and all fat research focused on this omega-6 fat. The omega-3 series of fats was not considered, and the discovery of their many derived compounds (such as eicosanoids and docosanoids) was in its initial state. The relationship of EPA and DHA deficiencies to increased ischemic heart disease (IHD) was unknown. Over the years, interest in the health benefits of consuming omega-3 LC-PUFAs, EPA and DHA, has also been aimed at the intake of ALA.

The focus of interest has been twofold: whether ALA has health benefits of its own and whether the conversion of ALA to longer-chained omega-3 fatty acids in humans is sufficient to produce desirable levels of EPA and DHA.

Health Benefits of ALA

Despite years of additional studies and research on the issue, the Institute of Medicine states, "Alpha-linolenic acid is [still] not known to have any specific functions other than to serve as a precursor for synthesis of EPA and DHA." Heart health, as Dr. Dyerberg was soon to discover, involves more than the old concept of EFAs. What is important to heart health goes beyond proper growth and development and far beyond the classical symptoms of EFA deficiency of scaly skin and excessive thirst. Cardiovascular optimization involves the LC-PUFAs, EPA and DHA. The only fatty acids known for cardiovascular optimization are EPA and DHA.

Heart Health and Good Health Demand More EPA and DHA Than ALA Can Supply

Plants are the most common source of ALA. Plants can introduce new double bonds between an existing double bond and the terminal methyl group and thus form omega-3 PUFAs. Humans and other animals cannot create omega-3 PUFA. They can, however, lengthen mid-chain PUFAs into LC-PUFAs and can even add a double bond or two—but on a very limited basis. The body is very inefficient in producing either EPA or DHA from plant-based sources of ALA such as flaxseeds or from stearidonic acid (SDA), another omega-3 LC-PUFA having a carbon chain length of eighteen and containing four double bonds. SDA is a metabolic intermediate in the conversion process of ALA to EPA. SDA is present in some seaweeds, the oils of borage, currants and echium, and certain fish. SDA is better converted into EPA than is ALA, but the body is still not capable of converting enough SDA into EPA for optimal needs.

We mentioned earlier that the conversion of ALA to EPA and DHA in the body is slow and limited. As noted, some animals (including humans) have enzymes that can add double bonds and lengthen the fatty acid (desaturation and elongation) in PUFAs, but not after the omega-9 position in the fatty acid. Humans and other animals can increase unsaturation to a very limited extent, but can't change an omega-6 into an omega-3, nor can they make omega-6 or omega-3 fatty acids.

High levels of LA in the Western diet further inhibit the low rate of ALA conversion in humans. In addition, the body can form a small amount of EPA and even a lesser amount of DHA from ALA due to the large proportion of dietary ALA that is oxidized during metabolism. (Oxidation is a natural process that occurs when fats are exposed to oxygen, creating free radicals, which damage cells.) Because of its limited conversion of omega-3 fatty acids in the body, ALA contributes only a little to the heart health benefits attributed to EPA and DHA, since only about 1–5 percent of ingested ALA becomes EPA and next to nothing of DHA.

Even ALA supplementation does not result in appreciable accumulation of omega-3 LC-PUFAs in plasma. It modestly raises EPA and a negligible amount of DHA. To obtain desirable levels of omega-3 LC-PUFAs by supplementation, far lower and dietary acceptable doses are effective when supplementing with such preformed (already formed from EPA and DHA) fatty acids as fish oil-based supplements, than by taking the precursor ALA. Obtaining desirable heart health benefits with ALA intake would necessitate eating a nearly vegan (meat- and dairy-free) diet and consuming an impractical amount of flaxseed oil!

For these reasons, you can see why it is difficult to consume enough ALA to raise EPA and DHA levels in the body either by diet or supplementation. Even if very high amounts of ALA and very little LA are consumed, the conversion of ALA to EPA and DHA can be enhanced, but it will still fall short of what is required for optimization of heart health. This is why the diet of the Eskimos was protective against heart disease and the diets in Western nations were not; this is the why Eskimos don't get heart attacks and Westerners do.

To prevent IHD, one should focus on EPA and DHA. Our focus is on optimization and not merely deficiency. The state of knowledge and consensus of experts in the field are that ALA's conversion to EPA and DHA is too inefficient to rely on for optimum heart health. Most scientists in the field agree and note that the most recent studies confirm the lower range of conversion (more toward 1 percent than 5 percent) among those consuming standard Western diets. A 2001 study using radioisotopes to follow the conversion found: "Only about 0.2 percent of the plasma alpha-linolenic acid was destined for synthesis of EPA" (Plourde, 2001).

Even if the conversion is many times higher in some people, whatever the percentage is, it isn't enough to produce the heart benefits produced by EPA and DHA. One percent or 5 or 10 percent is not 100 percent! If ALA did produce sufficient amounts of EPA and DHA, there would have been no need for Dr. Dyerberg to go to Greenland and find EPA and DHA in the blood of the Eskimos. There would have been ample EPA and DHA in most people's blood from ALA in their diets, and people would have only 10 percent of the IHD.

This is not to say that ALA is of little value or that it produces no benefit. It is an EFA and the body relies on it to avoid the risk of deficiency. ALA is good and should be in everyone's diet, but it does not significantly contribute to the strong heart benefits of EPA and DHA, nor to the many other health benefits you'll read about in Part Two.

ALA Does Not Convert to DHA

Young healthy people consuming an ideal diet can convert some ALA into EPA and then a minimal fraction into DHA (Arterburn, 2006). Not only are our bodies very inefficient at converting ALA to EPA, but older adults are even more inefficient in making DHA from ALA than younger people. Pregnant women cannot meet the needs of the fetus for the healthy development of brain, retina, and nervous tissue without dietary DHA, even if pregnant women convert more ALA than non-pregnant do. In infants, however, very high amounts of ALA did result in some increase in blood DHA, as will be discussed in Chapter 10.

The International Society for the Study of Fatty Acids and Lipids (ISSFAL), a group made up of more than 500 scientists, published their official statement on ALA supplementation and conversion to LC-PUFAs in people in the peer-reviewed journal for experts in this field, *Prostaglandins, Leukotrienes and Essential Fatty Acids* (Brenna, 2009). The ISSFAL statement concludes, "With no other changes in diet, improvement of blood DHA status can be achieved with dietary supplements of preformed DHA, but not with supplementation of alpha-linolenic acid, EPA, or other precursors."

ALA supplementation can increase EPA slightly but not optimally. However, the evidence clearly shows that precursor supplementation does not increase blood levels of DHA whether the supplement is ALA, EPA, or SDA. The only means known for increasing blood DHA by supplementation in adults is through the consumption of preformed DHA.

LA CONVERSION TO AA

The enzymes needed to make EPA are monopolized by LA, as large amounts of LA are converted into AA. You may remember from our discussion in Chapter 2 that omega-6 PUFAs undergo an additional conversion process to cis fats. Cis LA is easily converted to AA when it is found in unheated, unprocessed vegetable oils. However, the process of conversion can be thwarted when these LA-rich oils undergo partial hydrogenation (a manufacturing process that utilizes high temperatures and catalysts to add hydrogen atoms). During the process, some of the cis LA is converted into trans fatty acids—fats you want to avoid.

Trans Fatty Acids

Trans fats are made up of trans fatty acids. Today, most Westerners consume diets that are low in natural, whole foods and are high in chemically altered foods. Many of these diets contain too much partially hydrogenated vegetable oil—a fractionated substance that is abundant in processed and packaged foods. These altered, man-made fats react far differently in the body than natural whole foods (see "Good Fats Gone Bad" on page 58).

The majority of natural LA-rich fats in processed foods have been altered by a process called hydrogenation. In that process, vegetable oil is forced to react under pressure with hydrogen gas at temperatures between 250° and 400° F for several hours in the presence of a catalyst such as nickel or platinum. Hydrogenation saturates unsaturated fatty acids in the oils with hydrogen. However, this industrial process cannot control where the hydrogen atoms are added to the unsaturated double bonds. Randomly adding hydrogen atoms to PUFAs converts natural food components into many compounds, some of which have never been eaten before by humans until these partially hydrogenated trans fats were manufactured. The purpose of hydrogenation is to solidify an oil so that it can be made to resemble real foods such as butter. The hydrogenation process imparts desirable features such as spreadability, texture, positive mouth feel, and increased shelf life to naturally liquid vegetable oils. But hydrogenation ruins the nutritional value of vegetable oils!

The human diet has always contained small amounts of trans fatty acids. Natural trans fats are found in the meat and dairy products from such grazing animals as cattle, sheep, goat, deer, buffalo, and antelope. Microorganisms in the animals' digestive tracts try to get rid of the PUFAs found in the plant foods eaten by these animals. Most ruminant fats have about 2–3 percent trans fatty acids, whereas partially hydrogenated vegetable fats are commonly 30–40 percent and as high as 50–60 percent in processed and packaged foods. Only recently has there been an official effort to lower the amount of trans fats in our diets. In the past, efforts to limit trans fats were dismissed by the processed foods industry, which tried to convince the public that trans fats were essentially the same as saturated fats.

GOOD FATS GONE BAD

The trans fatty acids found in nature are different from the trans fatty acids formed by people during the hydrogenation process. The major trans fatty acids in partially hydrogenated vegetable oils have their double bonds at different positions (carbon numbers) than natural trans fats. As an example, a trans fat having its trans double bond at the ninth carbon has been identified as a health problem by much research. (The common name given to the eighteen-carbon trans fatty acid having a trans conformation at the ninth carbon is elaidic acid.) Health questions about trans fats with their trans bonds at the tenth and twelfth carbons have also been raised. The trans fats with their trans double bonds at the ninth, tenth, and twelfth carbons usually make up half or more of the total trans isomers in partially hydrogenated vegetable oils. Partially hydrogenated oils make up to 50–60 percent of trans fatty acids!

In the early days of trans fatty acid research, researchers assumed that the trans fatty acids found in ruminant fats were no different than those produced by partial hydrogenation in the factory. But subsequent studies showed that the amount of trans fats in ruminant fats was actually much smaller than that in processed fats. It was also assumed that man-made trans fats had no different effect on the machinery in cell membranes than natural trans fats. Yet all studies of trans fats produced by partially hydrogenating vegetable oils have shown an adverse effect on cell machinery.

Trans Fats Impede Cell Function

Trans fats are shaped differently in space and are difficult for the body to process. The problem arises when a large number of the trans fatty acids are consumed from foods and are deposited in those parts of the cell membranes that are supposed to have either saturated fatty acids or cis unsaturated fatty acids; under these circumstances, the trans fatty acids essentially foul up the machinery.

A cell membrane consists of a double phospholipid layer that contains LC-PUFAs from both the omega-3 and omega-6 families. The membrane also contains cholesterol and saturated fatty acids to give a balance of rigidity to the flexible PUFA-containing phospholipids. Balance is the key. Insufficient EPA and DHA create a stiff membrane that does not function properly and the health of the cell is impaired.

Cell membranes are barriers that separate the working mechanism of the cell from its environment. Cell membranes selectively let in the nutrients the cell needs and let out the waste products it does not. Membranes also contain receptors that pass chemical messengers and other chemical information through the membrane. The health of the cell membrane determines the health of every cell, every tissue, and every organ in our bodies.

Basically, trans fatty acids cause alterations to numerous physiological functions of cell membranes that are critical for cell homeostasis, such as appropriate membrane transport and membrane fluidity. These fatty acid isomers can also produce alterations in adipose cell size, cell number, lipid class, and fatty acid composition, which can have deleterious effects.

Trans fatty acids disrupt cell function in part by their ability to inhibit the function of membrane-related enzymes such as desaturase, which results in decreased conversion of LA to AA and other omega-6 fats. Trans fatty acids also interfere with the necessary conversion of short- and medium-chain omega-3s to long-chain omega-3s, and escalate the adverse effects of essential fatty acid deficiency. This latter effect was shown especially by the work of Dr. Holman and his colleagues at the Hormel Institute in Minnesota; other adverse effects have been shown by many researchers, including lipid expert Dr. Mary Enig at the University of Maryland. Some of the adverse effects show that trans fatty acids:

- Decrease levels of testosterone in male animals, increase level of abnormal sperm, and interfere with gestation in females;

- Correlate to low birth weight in human infants;

- Lower the amount of cream volume in milk from lactating females in all species studied (including humans), thus lowering the overall nutritional quality available to the infant;

- Cause a dose-response decrease in visual acuity in infants to fourteen months of age who are fed human milk with increasing levels of trans fatty acids;

- Elevate bad LDL (low-density lipoprotein) cholesterol levels and lower good HDL (high-density lipoprotein) cholesterol;

- Raise the atherogenic lipoprotein(a) in humans, whereas saturated fatty acids lower lipoprotein (a);

- Affect immune defense by lowering efficiency of B cells, a white blood cell that produces antibodies;

- Decrease the response of the red blood cell to insulin, thus having a potentially undesirable effect in diabetics;

- Are linked to brain-volume shrinkage, which is associated with Alzheimer's disease risk;

- Potentiate free-radical formation and cause adverse alterations in the activities of the enzyme system that metabolizes chemical carcinogens and drugs.

EPA AND DHA ARE ESSENTIAL

Well, so much for the background on different types of fats. The important point to keep in mind is that there are different types of fats and that the right intake of each is needed for optimal health. Heart health requires that we consume adequate amounts of both omega-3 and omega-6 fatty acids but in the proper metabolic balance.

Unfortunately, through the past fifty years or more, our fatty acid intake has changed, leading to an overabundance of dietary omega-6 AA and the disappearance of dietary omega-3 EPA and DHA—the missing factors that are increasing our risks not only for heart disease but also for many diseases and disorders. Those of us with very high amounts of omega-6 AA already in our diets should consider reducing any excessive intake and increasing the amount of omega-3 EPA and DHA in our diets. This can be accomplished by increasing our intake of cold-water fatty fish like salmon, sardines, mackerel, and other dietary sources of EPA and DHA including supplements, while avoiding foods with trans fats and reducing any excessive omega-6 intake.

6

The Omega-3 Requirement

The take-home message of this book is that adequate amounts of the omega-3 long-chain polyunsaturated fatty acids (LC-PUFAs) are needed for optimal health. Unfortunately, through the past fifty years, the amount of omega-3 LC-PUFAs in Western diets has decreased considerably and at an ever-increasing pace. On average, the U.S. diet contains about 95 milligrams (mg) of EPA and DHA per day per person (80 mg for men and 110 mg for women). This is considerably short of the 500 mg per day needed for minimal heart health benefits that we will describe later in this book, and far short of the 1,000 mg per day that we recommend as a minimum for optimal health. Dietary surveys also point out that in 20 percent of U.S. citizens, the intake is close to zero!

As expected, the decrease of EPA and DHA in the diet has resulted in a decrease of EPA and DHA in the tissues. A study of fatty acid consumption during the twentieth century concludes, "The apparent increased consumption of LA [omega-6 linoleic acid], which was primarily from soybean oil, has likely decreased tissue concentrations of EPA and DHA during the twentieth century" (Blasbalg, 2011).

It is of utmost importance to begin by *increasing* the amount of EPA and DHA in our diets, but optimal health requires that we also reduce the amount of trans fatty acids in our diets.

WHAT HAS HAPPENED TO DIETARY OMEGA-3?

We now recognize that a balance of omega-3 and omega-6 fats that is close to the balance of fats in the Paleolithic diets, which humans ate for many thousands of years, is a better fit for our genetic makeup than more recent agricultural diets and modern fast-food diets. Through the millennia the human diet has undergone four major transformations. With each dietary shift, the amount of omega-6 fats consumed has increased, and the amount of omega-3 fats has decreased. The ratio of omega-6 to omega-3 fats typical of each dietary era are indicated in parentheses:

- Caveman Diet (1:1)

- Agricultural Revolution Diet (4:1)

- Industrial Revolution Diet (10:1)

- Convenience/Fast-Food Diet (14–25:1)

It is important to remember that the Eskimos studied by Dr. Dyerberg in the 1970s not only consumed a diet high in omega-3 EPA and DHA, but they only had about one-half the omega-6 fatty acids in their diets as in typical Western diets.

Let's trace what has happened to the omega-3 content in our diets over the years. As people began to consume more foods containing omega-6 fatty acids, they tended to eat fewer foods with omega-3 fatty acids. One fat replaces another. It is not that omega-6 fatty acid foods are bad for us—after all, omega-6 fats are classified as essential fatty acids. It's that they tend to squeeze out omega-3 fatty acid foods, which are not as convenient to find. Additionally, there is more competition from the omega-6 fatty acids for the enzymes that elongate the short-chain omega-3 fatty acids into long-chain fatty acids.

Caveman Diet

Before the advent of agriculture about 10,000 years ago, primitive humans were hunter-gatherers. They hunted wild animals, fish, and birds for their meat and gathered berries, nuts, green leaves, and roots for their plant food. Of course, the ratio of animal to plant matter varied with geographic location, climate, and season; nonetheless, humans' intake of omega-3s and omega-6s was about equal. Until people began cultivating grains and livestock, they rarely if ever drank milk beyond mother's milk in infancy or ate grains.

Agricultural Revolution Diet

With the spread of agriculture, people shifted from nomadic groups to relatively stable and larger societies in order to tend fields. During this period people began consuming large amounts of grain, milk, and domesticated meat—and they became more sedentary as well. While their diet continued to contain large quantities of green leaves, which are rich in omega-3 fatty acids, the introduction of grains as a staple food, which is high in omega-6 fatty acids, shifted the balance of omega-6s to omega-3s to 4:1 ratio. The fatty acids in grains are predominantly omega-6s, which shift the eicosanoid balance more toward inflammatory activity.

Industrial Revolution Diet

With the industrial revolution and the advent of grain mills and sugar refineries, the human diet changed even more dramatically. Beginning around 1900, whole grains were routinely refined, removing the germs and husks and much of their content of omega-3 fats, B vitamins, and minerals, and consumption of refined sugar started to become commonplace. The machine age had the effect of forcing upon the people of the industrialized nations (especially the United States) a gigantic human feeding experiment. Terrestrial animals (such as beef, pork, mutton, and poultry) that we ate began to be increasingly fed corn or grain instead of natural grasses or brush. The addition of heavy presses made it possible to extract oils from plant seeds to make vegetable oils. Over the period from 1909 to 1999, soybean oil, which contains a high percentage of LA and a modest percentage of ALA, became the largest contributor of both LA and ALA to the U.S. diet, accounting for more than two-thirds of the edible oil consumed and shifting the balance of omega-6s to omega-3 to 10:1.

Convenient/Fast-Food Diet

As modern food-processing techniques increased the availability of packaged convenience foods—the plasticizing of real food into pseudo-foods by increasing their shelf life via partial hydrogenation—the balance of fatty acids was dramatically affected once again. Today's full panoply of diets—from fast-food burgers to varying concepts of balanced diets and food groups—bears little resemblance, superficially or in actual nutritional constituents, to the diverse, lean-meat, plant-based, whole-food diet that our primitive ancestors consumed over millions of years. For example, today, our fatty acid profile is substantially different from that of our ancient diet (1:1 vs. 14–25:1). In other words, our present-day diet fails to provide the biochemical and molecular requirements of Homo sapiens.

Essentially, food processing has all but depleted the amount of omega-3 fatty acids in our diets. Because omega-3 fatty acids oxidize very readily, foods containing these highly oxidizable fatty acids can turn rancid quickly and be rejected by the consumer. One way to keep a food fresh longer on the shelf is to reduce its content of omega-3 fats. Omega-3 LC-PUFAs have stability or shelf life only about one-tenth as long as the same foods that contain omega-6s, making omega-3s incompatible with processed foods.

Using the hydrogenation process, food producers have learned how to purposely pressurize omega-6 oils like safflower, sunflower, soy, and corn oils to give them a longer and more stable shelf life. Omega-6 oils are used extensively in processed and packaged foods. As foods containing the more stable omega-6 fatty acids became more available, people chose them for convenience. The process of hydrogenating oils, however, destroys omega-3s and changes many omega-6s into harmful trans fats.

Another factor that has exacerbated the problem is the current low-fat dietary craze, which reduces the amount of all fats in the diet. Reducing the total amount of fat readily leads to decreasing the amount of EPA and DHA in the diet below that required for optimal health.

THE DEMISE OF OMEGA-3 AND THE RISE OF INFLAMMATION

As we discussed in Chapter 4, omega fatty acids are the nutrient precursors to eicosanoids, a group of hormonelike substances found in cell membranes that act as messengers and regulators of inflammation. Omega-6 fatty acids produce the chemical messengers that promote inflammation. Once inflammation becomes chronic, it leads to low-grade inflammation throughout the body that in turn can lead to many serious health problems. Omega-3 fatty acids, on the other hand, produce the chemical messengers that reduce inflammation. A metabolic balance of both is needed.

This disappearance of omega-3 fatty acids from Western diets is thought to play a major role in the emergence of many of our modern illnesses such as heart disease, high blood pressure, stroke, and Alzheimer's disease. As the omega-3 content in our diet was decreasing, the incidence of these degenerative diseases—which were at that time thought to be due to aging and are now considered largely due to low-grade inflammation—began increasing. Even though the dietary ratio had changed somewhat before modern times, omega-3 fatty acids had been able to keep this low-grade, smoldering inflammation in check.

In addition to the detrimental effects that a diet lacking in omega-3 fatty acids has on the production of anti-inflammatory eicosanoids, the lack of omega-3s results in changes in the cell membrane. Omega-3s are responsible for the fluidity of cell membranes. As the fatty acid composition of the membrane shifts toward having fewer LC-PUFAs and/or more saturated fatty acids, it causes these cell membranes to become more rigid. Scientists have now learned these nutritional changes compromise the behavior of membranes in all cells in the body and thus negatively affect the health of all cells.

A Western Deficiency

By 1985 it was becoming apparent to scientists that the amount of omega-3 intake in the typical Western diet was so low that it was considered a deficiency. There was also evidence that in many, and perhaps most diets, omega-6 intake might be higher than optimum. In 1986 Dr. Dyerberg participated in an important conference of scientists arranged by a consortium, including the National Institutes of Health (NIH), the National Fisheries Institute, and the Department of Commerce in Washington,

D.C. The conference was on the Health Effects of Polyunsaturated Fatty Acids in Seafood.

Many of the attending scientists were already aware that a huge problem existed due to diets being deficient in the omega-3s, especially EPA and DHA. As scientists from around the world presented their evidence of various aspects of the problem, and as the total picture unfolded, it became clear that most modern diets lacked sufficient quantities of omega-3 fatty acids to make the desired levels of eicosanoids and the proper balance of eicosanoids needed for optimal health.

Many scientists at the conference concluded that a metabolic balance of omega-3 and omega-6 fatty acids was crucial and proposed *increasing* dietary omega-3 intake. Other scientists proposed *balancing* dietary omega-3 and omega-6 intake by consuming the appropriate ratios of each group. Their rationale was that because the excess of omega-6s was depleting the supply of enzymes needed to make long-chain omega-3s, which are required for eicosanoid formation, this rendered the sparse omega-3s in the diet of little use because they could not effectively compete for these needed enzymes. As a result, the unfavorable ratio of omega-6s over omega-3s in the diet prevented the body from making the balance of eicosanoids needed for optimal health.

The conference presented the scientists with new and different ideas to focus on in their future research. It is our view that both omega-3s and omega-6s are critical and that the problem with most diets in our Western culture today is that they are deficient in EPA and DHA. It is also our view that the "balance" concept has not been adequately verified under "real life" conditions and that balancing fatty acid intake is difficult and impractical. It is proven that restoring EPA and DHA to adequate levels will help bring about the health benefits we discuss in this book. However, the most critical factor is to *increase* dietary EPA and DHA.

This tactic is well supported by the body of science. At this writing, we consider it difficult for the general public to determine for themselves what their total intake of omega-6 and omega-3 fatty acids is, and it is impractical to suggest dietary guidelines based on ratios alone. Blood tests, such as the omega-3 index (which we will discuss in Chapter 8 on heart disease), may provide reliable guidance in determining one's dietary intake of omega-3 and omega-6 PUFAs. First things first: Be sure to get the recommended amounts of EPA and DHA.

Let's review the causes of the disappearance of omega-3 fatty acids from the typical Western diet:

1. With the availability of packaged convenience foods, foods high in omega-3-fatty acids such as fish and seafood are being eaten less often.

2. Partial hydrogenation of oils destroys omega-3s and increases undesirable trans fats.

3. Omega-3 fats are purposely removed from processed foods to give them a longer shelf life.

4. Many people are eating a low-fat diet to control their weight and body fat, which lowers all fats, including omega-3 EPA and DHA.

All total, these dietary factors have drastically reduced our intake of omega-3 fatty acids. As a result, our health has declined, and many inflammation-related diseases are now epidemic. We are a nation nutritionally deficient in omega-3 LC-PUFAs.

OPTIMAL REQUIREMENTS

As mentioned at the beginning of this chapter, in the United States the average daily intake of EPA plus DHA is 95 mg. In 20 percent of U.S. citizens, the intake is close to zero! The minimum recommended intake is 400–600 mg a day. However, as we will discuss in later chapters, this is considerably short of the recommended daily intake of EPA and DHA to protect against heart disease (1,000 mg); to reduce triglycerides (3,000 mg); to support the healthy development of the brain, retina, and nervous in the fetus and infant (300 mg); and to maintain optimal health (1,000 mg). It is important both to obtain adequate amounts of omega-3 and omega-6 PUFAs in the diet, and consequently a proper ratio between the anti-inflammatory eicosanoid/docosanoid and pro-inflammatory eicosanoid/docosanoid families.

In Part Two of this book, we will examine the evidence showing that increasing EPA/DHA intake reduces our risk of many common diseases.

We will start with heart disease in Chapter 8. But first, let's see how Dr. Dyerberg's pioneering research fit together with research from several other scientists.

Research Gains Interest and Acceptance by Other Scientists

nitially, the findings from Dr. Dyerberg and his team of researchers were not widely recognized for two reasons: First, those who had been fixated on dietary cholesterol as the only risk factor in heart disease dismissed the team's findings as irrelevant because the studies were done on Eskimos. And, second, some of the group's initial research had been published in European journals and was not readily available in all libraries worldwide. Remember, this was the 1970s before the Internet. Scientists had to have hard copies of expensive subject-specific journals or had to attend applicable conferences in order to exchange information. Abstract services were in rudimentary stages, and it was difficult to disseminate information across disciplines.

WORD SPREADS

The danger of focusing on only one risk factor—no matter how strong or weak—is that other potentially important factors are ignored. However, increasingly, other scientists expanded on Dyerberg's research and the word spread. Many other scientists, including me, became very interested. In fact, I became very excited. Until this point, I had found Dr. Dyerberg's research very enlightening, but with the additional information brought forth in 1980, I found it to be compelling. The highlights of Dr. Dyerberg's initial research findings during the 1970s and early '80s are summarized in Table 7.1 (on the following page).

TABLE 7.1. SUMMARY OF DYERBERG RESEARCH FINDINGS, 1971–1980	
YEAR	RESEARCH FINDING
1971	Observed two unidentified peaks "X" and "Y" in Eskimo blood
1975	Identified compounds in blood as EPA and DHA
1975	Found EPA and DHA in other populations
1977	Hypothesized relationship between blood levels of EPA and DHA and blood clotting
1979	Confirmed effect of EPA and DHA on blood clotting
1980	Confirmed high blood levels of EPA and DHA are related to Eskimo diet

Our Common Points of Interest

Concurrently with the publication of Dr. Dyerberg's research, I was publishing articles and books examining the inconsistencies in the dietary
cholesterol theory. It's important to note that it was *dietary* cholesterol
not *blood* cholesterol levels I was questioning.

While conducting research on antioxidants (compounds that help
protect the body from harmful free radicals) and heart disease, I had
observed that the dietary cholesterol theory just didn't fit all the facts.
Proof of a theory is not like a sports game, where the outcome is decided
by a majority of points. A scientific theory needs only one aspect that
doesn't hold true to be totally invalid. It's either all or nothing. Either the
theory is correct in all aspects or it is incorrect. I was calling attention
to the flaws in the dietary cholesterol theory. Yes, some facts did fit the
theory, but the requirement is that *all* facts must fit the theory. Half-
truths and wishful thinking don't make a theory a fact. In my opinion,
the dietary cholesterol-heart disease theory is filled with premises that
have repeatedly been proven false. As Dr. Dyerberg and his colleagues
were finding, even blood LDL-cholesterol was not a perfect indicator of
heart disease risk. Heart disease has several facets and independent risk
factors. The Dyerberg group was finding that blood EPA/DHA levels
trumped blood cholesterol in terms of predicting heart disease risk. As
we will discuss in the next chapter, a new risk indicator based on blood

EPA/DHA levels is a more accurate indicator of heart disease risk and is now gaining acceptance.

My point here is not whether you choose to subscribe to the dietary cholesterol theory—that's your personal choice and it really doesn't impact the fact that dietary EPA and DHA dramatically affect heart disease and other modern disorders. I mention it here only because it explains how the research of Dr. Dyerberg was brought to my attention and why I came to write the first book ever published on fish oil. Heart disease, as research has shown, is a multifaceted, complex illness. At that time, Dr. Dyerberg's observations fit a new theory of heart disease, one that challenged the role of dietary cholesterol. The fact that Eskimos eat a high-cholesterol, animal-fat diet, and at the time of Dr. Dyerberg's study were virtually free of heart disease, proved other factors were at play. When Dr. Dyerberg's and his colleagues' research was recognized as a "nutrition classic," the editor of the *Lancet* stated the following:

> Editor's note: These early observations by Bang et al were crucial in formulating a hypothesis to account for the low incidence of coronary heart disease in a population consuming a high-fat, high-cholesterol diet (1971).

Readers can take advantage of these findings concerning EPA and DHA regardless of what other heart-disease strategies they wish to utilize. Why put all your eggs in one basket? (Pun intended.) For clarification, note that we are referring to the cholesterol content of our *diet*. We do not in any way dispute the risk to some associated with high *blood* cholesterol as measured by the cholesterol lipoprotein carrier, LDL cholesterol. This is an accepted risk factor for heart disease, but it is not the most reliable risk predictor. Other independent risk factors should be considered as well. The truth is, however, that the cholesterol in our diet has only a minor influence on blood cholesterol level.

The findings of Dr. Dyerberg and his team complemented my own; our research and approach to diet and heart disease now had a point of common interest.

Introducing the Public to EPA and DHA

In 1972, about the time when Dr. Dyerberg identified two unknown compounds in Eskimo blood, I published an article on my research in *American Laboratory* magazine entitled "Dietary Cholesterol: Is It Related to Serum Cholesterol and Heart Disease?" In 1977 I expanded this research into a book called *Supernutrition Against Heart Disease.* Since heart disease is a multifaceted illness involving several risk factors, this book looked at the many aspects of diet and heart disease.

Perhaps it was these publications that encouraged other scientists to bring Dr. Dyerberg's research to my attention. The role of platelet aggregation (sticking together of blood platelets) and blood viscosity (thickness of blood) in heart disease made a lot of sense to me and fit well with my findings of antioxidant research. You don't just have a myocardial infarction (death of heart tissue) unless you have a blood clot. Keeping the blood slippery and free from clotting will reduce the probability of having the common heart attack, also called an acute myocardial infarction (AMI or MI).

One scientist in particular furthered my interest in Dr. Dyerberg's research. That scientist was Dr. Tom Sanders, a professor of nutrition at Queen Elizabeth College in London. Dr. Sanders visited my laboratory here in the United States, where he shared some of his work that was in the process of publication. Sanders published his research on the effects of fish oil supplements on blood platelets in the *British Journal of Nutrition* in 1981.

The research of Dr. Dyerberg, Dr. Sanders, and other scientists inspired me to write the first book on fish oils called *EPA—Marine Lipids: In the Battle Against Heart Disease, an Answer Comes From the Sea.* This book, which I wrote for the general public, was published in 1982 and was based on the thirty published studies of the time. The book quickly and widely brought Dr. Dyerberg's and his colleagues research to the public and encouraged the introduction of commercial fish oil supplements. I was pleased that the book helped introduce fish oil to many people and helped improve their health.

Growing Acceptance by Scientists

As increasing numbers of scientists picked up on Dr. Dyerberg's research, the number of scientific publications reporting on the topic began rapidly increasing. In 1987 I published a booklet called *Fish Oil Update* to inform the public about the latest EPA/DHA research related to arthritis, diabetes, migraines, and some forms of cancer, as well as heart disease. In the intervening five years, the number of published scientific articles had grown tenfold.

As you can see from Figure 7.1, the number of published scientific

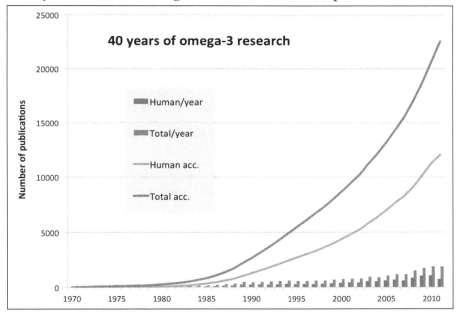

Figure 7.1. Forty years of omega-3 research. The smooth curves represent the number of accumulated total publications over the years, with the blue line representing the human studies and the red line representing all studies. The bars represent the number of studies in the year beneath the bars, with the blue bar representing the number of human studies and the red bar representing all studies.

articles on EPA and DHA has grown exponentially. Now, with over 20,000 studies, of which more than 12,000 are human clinical trials, EPA and DHA are two of the most researched substances in modern medicine.

The acceptance of Dr. Dyerberg's and colleagues' research is exemplified by the fact that the *Lancet*, a leading medical journal, has reprinted two of their reports—"Plasma lipid and lipoprotein pattern in Greenlandic west-coast Eskimos" (1971) and "Hæmostatic function and platelet polyunsaturated fatty acids in Eskimos" (1979)—with the designation of "nutrition classic." By the end of 2011, yet another report in the *Lancet* had been cited more than 1,300 times by other scientists in their reports: "Eicosapentaenoic acid and prevention of thrombosis and atherosclerosis" (1978). Table 7.2 lists the most frequently cited of the 300 publications by Dr. Dyerberg.

TABLE 7.2. CITATION CLASSICS OF DR. JØRN DYERBERG (AS OF DECEMBER 2011)	
NUMBER OF TIMES CITED	ARTICLE TITLE AND PUBLICATION
1,308	Dyerberg J, Bang HO, Stoffersen E, et al. "Eicosapentaenoic acid and prevention of thrombosis and atherosclerosis." *Lancet* 1978;2:117–119
755	Dyerberg J, Bang HO. "Hæmostatic function and platelet polyunsaturated fatty acids in Eskimos." *Lancet* 1979;2:433–435
620	Bang HO, Dyerberg J, Hjørne N. "The composition of food consumed by Greenland Eskimos." *Acta Medica Scandinavica* 1976;200:69–73
537	Dyerberg J, Bang HO, Hjørne N. "Fatty acid composition of the plasma lipids in Greenland Eskimos." *American Journal of Clinical Nutrition* 1975;28:958–966
425	Bang HO, Dyerberg, J, Nielsen AB. "Plasma lipid and lipoprotein pattern in Greenlandic west-coast Eskimos." *Lancet* 1971;1:1143–1146
394	Bang HO, Dyerberg J. "Plasma lipids and lipoproteins in Greenlandic west-coast Eskimos." *Acta Medica Scandinavica* 1972;192:85–94
389	Bang HO, Dyerberg J, Sinclair HM. "The composition of the Eskimo food in north western Greenland." *American Journal of Clinical Nutrition* 1980;33:2657–2661
291	Dyerberg J. "Linolenate-derived polyunsaturated fatty acids and prevention of atherosclerosis." *Nutrition Reviews* 1986;44:125–134

As far as the growing acceptance of Dr. Dyerberg's findings, in 2007 he was honored by the American Heart Association (AHA) in "Recognition of Outstanding Scientific Contribution for the Advancement of Heart

Health Worldwide." In 2008 he received the American Dietetic Association Foundation's Edna and Robert Langholz International Nutrition Award for his contribution to the international community in the field of nutrition. In 2011 a review of the relationship between EPA and DHA in the *New England Journal of Medicine* described the pioneering research of Drs. Dyerberg and Bang (De Caterina, 2011) this way:

> In a seminal article in 1978, Dyerberg and colleagues presented the hypothesis that marine ω–3 [omega-3] fatty acids might provide protection against atherosclerosis and thrombosis, and they began research on the potential effects of ω–3 fatty acids in the prevention and treatment of vascular disease.

The review concluded,

> On the basis of currently available evidence, the American Heart Association (AHA) has recommended that all adults eat fish (particularly fatty fish) at least twice a week, as well as vegetables containing plant-derived ω–3 fatty acids (ALA). The AHA also suggests that patients with documented coronary heart disease consume approximately 1 gram (1,000 mg) of EPA and DHA (combined) per day, from oily fish or fish-oil capsules (after consultation with a physician). The AHA recommendations also state that EPA/DHA supplements may be useful in patients with severe high triglyceride levels (>500 mg of triglycerides per deciliter), for whom effective doses are higher: 2 to 4 grams of EPA plus DHA per day to lower triglyceride levels by 20 to 40 percent.

Dr. Dyerberg considers himself privileged to have been a co-initiator of such an important science.

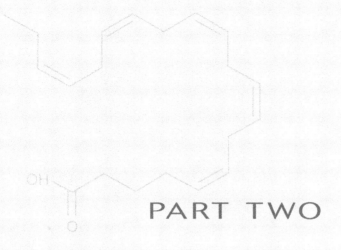

PART TWO

EPA and DHA at Work: Clinical Trials

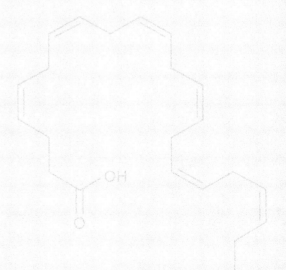

8

Heart Disease

You now have some history of how fish oil was discovered to help prevent heart attacks, as well as some basic biochemistry to help you better understand how the unique chemical structure of EPA and DHA give them this unique benefit. You really don't have to understand why. The bottom line is: EPA and DHA reduce the incidence and risk of heart disease. That's all you really have to know! Our objective is to help you improve your health and live better longer, and we believe—and science supports—that EPA and DHA can help you do that.

Here in Part Two, we let the facts speak for themselves as we present the latest clinical research on EPA and DHA and the evidence supporting their effectiveness at reducing the incidence and risk of our most common diseases and disorders. For example, studies have found that EPA and DHA can reduce your chance of dying a sudden death by 45 percent if you have a heart disease (GISSI, 1999; Albert, 2002)! One clinical study has shown that EPA and DHA can reduce your risk of dying from sudden cardiac death by 90 percent (Leon, 2008). Another study has found that DHA may reduce your chance of developing Alzheimer's disease by 45–50 percent (Schaefer, 2006). There is even credible evidence that EPA and DHA can help you stay younger longer (Farzaneh-Far, 2010)! Clinical studies have shown that these omega-3, long-chain polyunsaturated fatty acids (LC-PUFAs) can reduce the inflammation and pain of rheumatoid arthritis and the pain of osteoarthritis arthritis and other inflammatory diseases (Galarraga, 2008; Fritsch, 2010). No other nutritional measure—neither the addition of a nutrient nor the avoidance of a food component such as cholesterol—have produced results anywhere near this dramatic![1]

LOWER RISK OF HEART DISEASE
WITH HIGHER INTAKE OF EPA/DHA

Like most disease, heart disease is multifaceted and involves many aspects including genetics, behavioral, environmental, and lifestyle factors, as well as nutritional factors. EPA and DHA are not magic nutrients that can completely protect everyone from all risks for heart disease. Nor can EPA and DHA substitute for other essential nutrients needed for the cardiovascular system. However, many, if not most, people can have their risks of heart disease significantly reduced and postponed with adequate nourishment of EPA and DHA.

In science, we can study how nutrients and drugs affect groups of people better than we can study how they affect individuals. Each of us is unique—even biologically. This concept has long been recognized as *biochemical individuality.* More recently, we have been able to study the interactions of nutrients with individuals as the science of *nutrigenomics,* and the interactions of drugs and individuals as *pharmacogenomics.* The interactions go both ways—nutrients affect whether or not a nutrient activates an individual's genes and genes affect how an individual responds to a nutrient. Our genes provide a genetic blueprint, but our diet determines whether or not certain genes are activated or lie dormant. Thus, even though our family history provides clues to our possible risks for disease, we are not limited to the genes we inherited. We can choose lifestyle and dietary patterns that can very often override our inherited genes.

---

1. In Chapter 2 we mentioned that this book would focus on omega-3, long-chain, polyunsaturated fatty acids (LC-PUFAs), specifically EPA and DHA. Throughout Part Two when we discuss specific research studies, you will find that sometimes the researchers have investigated the actions of only specific PUFAs, such as EPA or DHA or both. At other times, the researchers may have investigated larger groups of PUFAs, such as all omega-3 PUFAs (not just EPA and/or DHA), and occasionally they may have studied all PUFAs, including all omega-3s and omega-6s. We have taken care to identify the specific type of fatty acid(s) the researchers studies, which may appear confusing to some readers at first.

Clinical studies are best done with large groups of individuals in order to average out the genetic and lifestyle variances of individuals. As a consequence, the results speak more to the group than to any particular individual within that group. As scientists, we prefer to be in the group with the lesser risk of a disease. We think you want to be in this lower risk group too. So, there are no guarantees, but we will describe several clinical studies that point to lower risk of heart disease with higher intakes of EPA and DHA.

Note: For ease of understanding throughout this chapter, we will mostly use the common term *heart disease* to cover various forms of cardiovascular diseases when we can do so without distorting the meaning of the data. Where it is critical to refer precisely to a specific form of a cardiovascular disease, we will do so. The terms used for various forms of cardiovascular disease have evolved through the years and in different countries, but commonly and generically, people prefer to consider them as heart disease. See the inset below for a glossary of common heart disease terms.

HEART DISEASE GLOSSARY

Acute coronary syndromes (ACS). An umbrella term for a group of diseases that can lead to reduced blood flow in the coronary arteries and cause ischemia (see below) or infarct.

Acute myocardial infarction (AMI) or myocardial infarction (MI). These are the terms most often used by physicians to identify what most nonprofessionals commonly call a heart attack. This term refers to the death (infarct) of heart tissue (myocardium).

Acute myocardial ischemia (AMI). Essentially another name for acute myocardial infarction.

Angina or angina pectoris. A condition (syndrome) characterized by sudden, severe, constricting pain below the sternum, most easily precipitated by exertion or excitement and caused by ischemia of the heart muscle, usually due to a coronary artery disease, such as arteriosclerosis.

Arteriosclerosis. Degenerative changes in the arteries, characterized by thickening of the vessel walls and accumulation of calcium with consequent loss of elasticity and lessened blood flow.

Atherosclerosis. A common form of arteriosclerosis in which fatty substances form a deposit of plaque within arterial walls.

Cardio. Heart.

Cardiovascular disease (CVD). Any disease affecting the heart and blood vessels.

Congestive heart failure. A condition in which the heart can no longer pump enough blood to the rest of the body.

Coronary artery disease (CAD). Also called coronary heart disease. A disease, such as atherosclerosis, affecting the arteries that supply blood directly to the heart.

Ischemia. A deficiency of blood supply and the oxygen carried by blood, which is produced by vasoconstriction or local obstacles to the arterial flow.

Ischemic heart disease (IHD). Also called ischemic cardiomyopathy. A deficiency of blood supply to the heart causing muscle damage.

Myopathy. Muscle damage or disease.

Clinical Studies

As one large study showed, the risk of dying prematurely from all causes of death is reduced by as much as 85 percent by maintaining optimal levels of EPA and DHA. Although this 2008 study was intended to primarily investigate the effect of EPA and DHA on atrial fibrillation (a common irregular heart rhythm), the researchers found that EPA and DHA levels were associated with an 85 percent reduction in premature deaths from any and all causes (Macchia, 2008). In 2009 another study showed similar results in heart attack survivors. Patients with the highest levels of EPA and DHA in their bodies were protected against any and all causes of death, not just heart-related conditions (Lee, 2009). The following year, another study of high-risk cardiovascular patients found a 47 percent reduction in risk from all causes. Clinical studies have many variables and differences in protocol, as well as differences in the severity of disease in the patients—so it is not surprising that the numbers jump around. What is important is that the body of science shows a consistent trend or pattern (Einvik, 2010).

The good news is that the protection provided by EPA and DHA can be experienced fairly quickly, even at young ages. In a Danish study of young women, ages fifteen to forty-seven, those who rarely or never ate fish had 50 percent more cardiovascular problems over eight years than those who ate fish regularly (Halldorsson, 2012). The study linked 48,627 women from the Danish National Birth Cohort to the Danish National Patients Registry for information on events of hypertensive, cerebrovascular, and ischemic heart disease used to define a combined measure of cardiovascular diseases. The study found that women who rarely or never ate fish faced a 90 percent higher risk of heart problems than those who ate fish weekly. When the researchers examined hospital admissions for cardiovascular disease, they found such admissions were three times higher among women who did not eat fish. The study concluded, "Our findings based on a large prospective cohort of relatively young and initially healthy women indicated that little or no intake of fish and omega-3 LC-PUFAs was associated with an increased risk of cardiovascular disease." Lead researcher, Dr. M. Strom, at the Centre for Fetal Programming at Statens Serum Institut in Copenhagen, noted that they saw a strong association with cardiovascular disease in the women who were still in their late thirties. For further reviews of the effects of fish oil on sudden cardiac death (the sudden cessation of heartbeat and cardiac function) and mortality, see the inset on the following page.

In this chapter we will discuss the heart health benefits of EPA and DHA and their ability to:

• Reduce risk of cardiovascular disease

• Reduce risk of sudden death from cardiovascular disease

• Protect against deposits in arteries

• Promote artery elasticity

• Promote a healthy, stable heartbeat

• Lower blood C-reactive protein (CRP) levels

• Lower blood triglyceride levels

• Lower blood pressure

REVIEWS WITH STRONG SUPPORTIVE EVIDENCE

The following articles provide excellent overviews of the effects of fish oil on sudden death from heart disease and mortality:

- "Towards Establishing Dietary Reference Intakes for Eicosapentaenoic and Docosahexaenoic Acids" by W. Harris, D. Mozaffarian, M. Lefevre, et al. *Journal of Nutrition* 2009;139(4):804S–819S.

- "Effect of Fish Oil on Arrhythmias and Mortality: Systematic Review" by H. Leon, M. C. Shibata, S. Sivakumaran, et al. *British Medical Journal* 2008;337:a2931.

- "Prevention of Sudden Cardiac Death with Omega-3 Fatty Acids in Patients with Coronary Heart Disease: A Meta-Analysis of Randomized Controlled Trials" by Y. T. Zhao, Q. Chen, X. Y. Sun, et al. *Annals of Medicine* 2009;41(4):301–310.

First Signs That EPA and DHA Do More Than Influence Blood Clotting

The first interest in EPA and DHA in preventing heart disease was how EPA reduced the risk of blood clots that result in heart attacks and strokes. Later, it was found that the major underlying cause of heart disease is uncontrolled inflammation in the wall of the arteries. During the inflammation process, plaques (commonly called cholesterol deposits) develop in the inflamed area. Inflammation within artery walls can interact and oxidize carriers of cholesterol in the blood called *low-density lipoprotein,* or LDL. The smaller and denser "pattern B" subgroup of LDL particles can contribute to plaque formation (in a role similar to that of an accomplice), but they themselves do not play a primary role or initiating role in this process. There are now suggestions that DHA can modify the more atherogenic LDL pattern B particles by changing them into the less dense and less atherogenic LDL pattern A particles (Bernstein, 2012). For more on cholesterol's role in heart disease, see the inset at right.

EPA and DHA reduce the inflammation and reduce the risk of developing plaques. A review of the science linking inflammation to atherosclerosis is presented by Dr. J. Keaney Jr. of the University of Massachusetts Medical School in the journal *Circulation* (Keaney, 2011).

A CHOLESTEROL PRIMER

Cholesterol is both a steroid and a lipid that is vital for cell membrane stabilization, producing sex hormones and vitamin D among other functions. Most cells can produce cholesterol themselves, but the body finds it more efficient to produce large quantities of cholesterol in the liver and then transport it to other cells. Since cholesterol is fat-like (a lipid), it is insoluble in blood, which is water-based. The body assembles particles containing both proteins and lipids called lipoproteins to transport fats and cholesterol in the blood. Major lipoproteins are classified as being high-density lipoproteins (HDL), low-density lipoproteins (LDL), intermediate-density lipoproteins (IDL), very low-density lipoproteins (VLDL), and chylomicrons.

LDL and HDL can carry cholesterol in their lipid interiors while their protein shells enable them to be carried in the bloodstream. LDL carries cholesterol to cells from the liver, while HDL returns unused cholesterol back to the liver. For decades, LDL has been referred to as the "bad cholesterol" and HDL as the "good cholesterol." However, recent research has found that it is not quite that simple as both LDL and HDL particles come in various sizes, composition, and densities that give them different properties.

There are several subclasses of lipoproteins of both LDL and HDL. The smaller, denser LDL lipoproteins are often called LDL pattern B particles particles whereas the fluffier, less dense LDL particles are often called LDL pattern A particles. The LDL pattern B lipoproteins penetrate easier into the arterial vessel wall and are more easily oxidized and able to become involved in the inflammatory damage within the artery walls than LDL pattern A lipoproteins (Bhalodkar, 2005).

The effectiveness of EPA and DHA has been evaluated against heart drugs including the statins such as Lipitor, and the combination of EPA and DHA were found to be more effective in reducing heart attacks and deaths (Studer, 2005).

New Risk Factor for Heart Disease

The scientific and medical communities now recognize that consuming omega-3 LC-PUFAs has significant benefits to the cardiovascular system. The relationship is so strong that a low level of omega-3 LC-PUFAs is now proposed as a risk factor for heart disease (Harris, 2009). The new risk factor is based on a measurement of fatty acid levels in red blood cells called the *omega-3 index,* and is expressed as a percentage of EPA and DHA of the total fatty acids. An omega-3 index of greater than 8 percent is the target cardioprotective level, based on the findings from several research studies. One of them reported that individuals with an average omega-3 index of 6.3 percent were 90 percent less likely to experience sudden cardiac death over a seventeen-year period compared to those with an index of less than 3.3 percent (Harris, 2008).

A growing number of scientific data suggest that this new indicator of risk is much more reliable than total cholesterol, LDL cholesterol, HDL cholesterol, triglycerides, homocysteine, and other blood risk predictors, including the new generation lipid tests for lipoprotein(a) [Lp(a)] and apolipoprotein B (ApoB), especially when it comes to predicting risk from sudden cardiac death (Harris, 2010).

An omega-3 index of greater than 8 percent is associated with a lower risk for acute coronary syndromes (ACS). ACS is an umbrella term used to cover any group of clinical symptoms compatible with acute myocardial ischemia or acute myocardial infarct. Acute myocardial ischemia is chest pain due to insufficient blood supply to the heart muscle that results from coronary artery disease.

The omega-3 index can discriminate among ACS patients and controls better than the standard risk factors (age, sex, smoking, cholesterol, HDL, blood pressure, and diabetes). A higher omega-3 index is associated with slowed "cellular aging" as measured by the five-year rate of telomere (the tips of DNA) shortening. (Cellular aging is discussed in detail in Chapter 16.)

Heart patients with below-average omega-3 index values die at a faster rate than those with above-average levels. Also, patients admitted to the hospital with a heart attack are less likely to develop ventricular arrhythmias if they have a higher versus a lower omega-3 index. In addition, inflammatory markers are inversely related to the omega-3 index.

The average value in the United States is around 4–5 percent, which can be compared to well over 8 percent in Japanese samples (Figure 8.1) and over 7 percent in a population in Barcelona, Spain. The Koreans also seem to have quite high levels. Japanese, Spanish, Norwegian, and Korean men have coronary heart disease death rates of 48, 92, 96, and

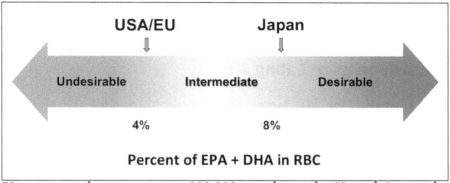

51, respectively, per year per 100,000 people; in the United States, the

Figure 8.1. Omega-3 index and risks of cardiovascular disease.

Data are from W. S. Harris, et al. and M. Itomura, et al.

rate is 153 deaths per 100,000.

Even a modest increase in EPA and DHA has produced amazing results. In a large multi-year clinical study, Dutch researchers reported a 62 percent lower risk of fatal heart attacks in people consuming a modest amount of EPA and DHA, approximately 230 milligrams a day (mg) per day, as compared with those consuming small amounts (approximately 40 mg) per day of EPA and DHA (de Goede, 2010).

A low dietary intake of omega-3 fatty acids and a high dietary intake of trans fatty acids are the dietary risks with the largest mortality effects in the United States. In the year 2005, 84,000 deaths in the United States were attributable to low omega-3 intake and 82,000 deaths to high trans fatty acid intake (Danaei, 2009).

INFLUENTIAL STUDIES OF CARDIAC EFFECTS

In several of the preceding chapters we have discussed how EPA and DHA help control blood stickiness or slipperiness by improving the balance of eicosanoids. Now, let's talk results. So many important studies show the heart health benefits of EPA and DHA. It's difficult to pick just a few to discuss, but let's home in on the clinical studies that caught the attention of many researchers and influenced the thinking of official organizations that make dietary recommendations and public policy.

Heart Benefits of Eating Fish

Let's start with the first large clinical study to examine the effect of increased intake of EPA and DHA on coronary heart disease (CHD): the 1989 Diet and Reinfarction Trial (DART). CHD is the nation's largest cause of premature death, killing more than 500,000 Americans each year. The DART study involved 2,033 men recovering from heart attack. They were randomly allocated to receive advice or to receive no advice on each of three dietary factors: an increase in fatty fish intake (or alternatively, a corresponding dose of fish oil supplements); a reduction in intake of certain fats (saturated fat) with an increase in others (PUFAs); or an increased intake of cereal fiber. The men advised to eat more fatty fish or to take the fish oil supplements had a 29 percent reduction in their two-year all-cause mortality compared with those in the two other groups who did not follow this advice. The other forms of advice did not have any significant effects on mortality (Burr, 1989).

The 1999 Gruppo Italiano per lo Studio della Sopravvivenza nell'Infarto miocardico (GISSI) Prevenzione Trial was the largest clinical study to examine the effect of increased intake of EPA and DHA on coronary heart disease. The GISSI-Prevention Trial randomized more than 11,300 people who had had a heart attack within two months of their enrollment into two groups. In one group, the subjects supplemented with 850 mg per day of EPA and DHA, while the control group took no supplement. In both groups the patients were treated with state-of-the-art cardiovascular medication. Follow-up three and a half years later found that the group taking the EPA/DHA supplement—at a dose slightly below that generally recommended for heart patients—showed a 21 percent reduction in total mortality compared with the control group. An analysis of the causes of death showed that among all cardiac causes, sudden cardiac death, which annually causes some 300,000 deaths in the United States, was the most positively affected by the omega-3 LC-PUFAs. It was reduced by 45 percent (GISSI, 1999)!

Figures 8.2–8.4 illustrate the consistent findings from three additional studies that add considerable support to the science showing EPA and DHA reduces the risk of death from cardiovascular disease. The most important message to note from these studies is that people who were in the top 25 percent of EPA/DHA combined intake have only between 10–20 percent of the cardiac risks of people in the bottom 25 percent of EPA/DHA intake. In each figure total EPA/DHA blood levels were measured and expressed with the omega-3 index.

In the 2008 study by R. C. Block, the blood content of EPA and DHA from 768 patients with ACS was measured and compared to 768 healthy controls, who were matched for age, sex, and race. The findings show that people with the highest content of EPA and DHA had the lowest risk of experiencing some form of cardiovascular disease. Figure 8.2 charts the EPA/DHA intake as three groupings: low

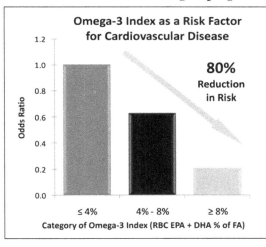

Figure 8.2.
The odds ratio of developing cardiovascular disease is inversely associated with the combined EPA/DHA content of the blood. *Data are from R. C. Block et al.; omega-3 index from W. S. Harris.*

(<4 percent), intermediate (4–8 percent), and high (>8 percent).

The data in Figures 8.3 and 8.4, from studies conducted by D. S. Siscovick and by C. M. Albert, show the relationships between blood levels of EPA and DHA and relative risk of sudden cardiac deaths.

In the 1995 Siscovick study, blood samples from 80 adults experiencing primary cardiac arrest and from 108 healthy matched controls were examined and compared. The subjects in the primary arrest group were not aware that they had heart disease at the time of their events. The findings showed that low blood levels of EPA and DHA were inversely associated with being in the cardiac arrest group (Siscovick, 1995). Figure 8.3 charts the EPA/DHA intake as four groupings: one grouping for each 25 percent (quartile) of omega-3 index. Each group is represented by a bar. As you can see, the risk of sudden cardiac death decreases linearly as the amount of EPA and DHA in the diet as measured by the percentage of EPA and DHA of all PUFAs contained in the red blood cells increases. The more EPA and DHA in the diet, the lower the risk of sudden cardiac death.

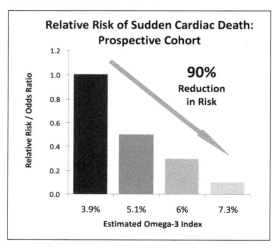

Figure 8.3.
Relationship between total EPA/ DHA content (expressed as the omega-3 index) and the risk for sudden cardiac death. *Data are from D. S. Siscovick et al.*

The first bar represents the group having blood levels of EPA and DHA in the lowest 25 percent, with an average omega-3 index of 3.9 percent. The incidence of cardiac death in this group is arbitrarily set at a risk of one, or 100 percent. The last bar (furthest to the right) represents the group having blood levels of EPA and DHA in the highest 25 percent, with an average omega-3 index of 7.3 percent. The risk of sudden cardiac death in this group is only 10 percent (a 90 percent reduction) of the risk of those in the first group with the omega-3 index of 3.9 percent. The middle bars represent the middle groupings of omega-3 index. They show that the risk decreases in a direct linear fashion as the average omega-3 index increases. (Sometimes a figure is worth a thousand words.)

In the 2002 Albert study, researchers looked at a patient cohort nested within the well-known Physicians' Health Study, which drew blood samples from 14,916 healthy male physicians for two years. Over the next seventeen years, ninety-four men experienced sudden cardiac death. In these cases, the EPA and DHA in previously drawn blood samples were compared to 184 matched controls (Albert, 2002). Figure 8.4 charts the EPA/DHA intake as four groupings as in Figure 8.3. As before, the bars show that the risk for death decreases as the omega-3 index increases.

In both this and the Siscovick study, those individuals with the highest EPA/DHA levels had only 10 percent the risk of sudden cardiac death of normal people compared with those who

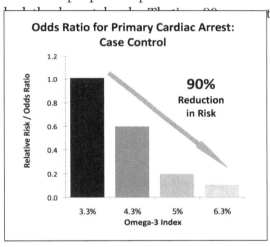

Figure 8.4.
Relationship between the total EPA and DHA (expressed as the omega-3 index) and sudden cardiac death.
Data are from C. M. Albert et al.

reduction! Later in the chapter, we will dis-
cuss the importance of EPA and DHA in normalizing heart rhythm and preventing abnormal heart rhythms that can lead to sudden cardiac death.

The obvious conclusion that can be drawn from these three figures is that EPA and DHA help prevent heart disease. Another conclusion worth noting is that Americans are deficient in nutritional omega-3 LC-PUFAs. As you may recall, in the United States, the average daily intake of EPA plus DHA is about 95 mg (Harris, 2009). A dietary study found that in 20 percent of U.S. citizens, the intake is close to zero (Dolecek, 1991)! Yet, the numbers might be even worse. The U.S. Department of Health & Human Services found when examining the U.S. population's intake of omega-3 fatty acids based on analyses of a single 24-hour dietary recall in NHANES III (a large national dietary survey), only 25 percent of Americans reported any amount of daily EPA or DHA intake (NHANES, 1999).

Heart Benefits of Fish Oil Supplements

In March 2006, an epidemiological study involving more than 30,000 people was reported at the 55th annual meeting of the American College of Cardiology by Dr. V. Raxwal and colleagues at the University of Kansas School of Medicine. Results from this study showed that the risk of dying was significantly reduced for people with coronary heart disease who had been taking fish oil supplements. The study found that if people were not taking the fish oil, they had a 2.96 times risk of dying compared with people who were taking the fish oil.

In their presentation, Raxwal and his colleagues reported that 2,870 patients taking fish oil supplements were followed from 1998 through 2005, along with 27,811 patients who were not taking fish oil supplements. During the seven-year study, 115 people who were taking the fish oil supplements died compared with 3,120 patients who had not been taking the capsules. Thus, about 11 percent of the patients not taking the fish oil died compared with 4 percent of those who were taking the fish oil supplements. That is a statistically significant difference. The study also examined patients who did not have coronary heart disease and compared them with patients who did, and found virtually the same relationship. Those who were not taking the supplements died at a greater rate than those taking omega-3 fatty acids. About 30 percent of those not taking fish oil supplements died compared to about 17 percent of those patients who were on fish oils. That difference was also statistically significant.

A negative finding from a large intervention study conducted in the Netherlands and reported in the *New England Journal of Medicine* (Kromhout, 2010) did not find any effect on ischemic heart disease at a dose nearly exactly that which had been used and produced amazing results in the Dutch study mentioned at the beginning of the chapter (de Goede, 2010). In the first study in patients who had had a heart attack and who were receiving state-of-the-art antihypertensive, antithrombotic, and lipid-modifying therapy, a low-dose supplementation with EPA and DHA (380 mg) per day did not significantly reduce the rate of major cardiovascular events. However, it should be noted that 380 mg is far lower than the typical dose now recommended for people with heart disease.

(In such patients the recommended dose is 1 gram of EPA and DHA per day.)

Despite the poor outcomes cited from several studies such as this, a study in *Current Atherosclerosis Reports* led by W. S. Harris points out that with each passing year the cardiovascular benefits of omega-3 fatty acids become clearer than ever (Harris, 2008). In their meta-analysis (a statistical syntheses) of six clinical studies, they found a significant dose-response relationship between the risk of dying from coronary heart disease and fish oil intake, with relative risk reductions of 37 percent at an average EPA/DHA intake of 566 mg per day. They suggested that research should be directed toward establishing minimum and optimal levels of EPA and DHA for reduction of heart disease risk.

Impact of Studies on Public Policy and Official Recommendations

What impact do these and hundreds of other studies have in respect to the total body of science on omega-3 and cardiovascular disease? Here is what the American Heart Association's (AHA) Nutrition Committee proclaimed in its official position paper published in 2002:

> Omega-3 fatty acids have been shown in epidemiological and clinical trials to reduce the incidence of CVD [cardiovascular disease]. . . . Large-scale epidemiological studies suggest that individuals at risk for CVD benefit from the consumption of plant- and marine-derived omega-3 fatty acids, although the ideal intakes presently are unclear. Evidence from prospective secondary prevention studies suggests that EPA and DHA supplementation ranging from 0.5 to 1.8 grams per day, either as fatty fish or supplements, significantly reduces subsequent cardiac and all-cause mortality.

This statement and supporting facts were approved by the AHA Science Advisory and Coordinating Committee on May 28, 2002, and published in great detail in their journal *Circulation* (2002). In the same journal in November of that year, the AHA published the Scientific Advisory's official recommendations for fish consumption, fish oil, omega-3 fatty acids, and heart disease (see Table 8.1).

TABLE 8.1. AHA SUMMARY OF RECOMMENDATIONS FOR OMEGA-3 FATTY ACID INTAKE

POPULATION	RECOMMENDATION
Patients without documented history of CHD	Eat a variety of (preferably oily) fish at least twice a week. Include in the diet oils and foods rich in ALA (flaxseed, canola, and soybean oils; flaxseeds; and walnuts).
Patients with documented history of CHD	Consume about 1 gram of EPA/DHA per day, preferably from oily fish. EPA/DHA supplements could be considered in consultation with a physician.
Patients with high triglycerides that need to be lowered	2–4 grams of EPA/DHA per day provided as capsules while under a physician's care.

Source: *Circulation* Nov 19, 2002;106(21):2747–2757

Several months later in the May 27, 2003 issue of *Circulation*, the AHA stated in a landmark editorial: "There is a need to consider a new indication for treatment with low dose omega-3 fatty acid or fish oil supplements—the prevention of cardiac death in patients with a prior heart attack."

However, we caution you that all fish are not equal and all methods of preparing fish are not protective. See the inset on fish preparation methods at right.

Two years later, the DHHS's Agency for Healthcare Research and Quality (AHRQ) also reviewed the evidence on omega-3s and cardio-vascular disease. The AHRQ report concluded:

Overall, the evidence from the primary and secondary prevention studies supports the hypothesis that consumption of omega-3 fatty acids (EPA, DHA, ALA[2]), fish, and fish oil reduces all-cause mortality and various CVD outcomes such as sudden death, cardiac death (coronary or MI death), and MI, although the evidence is strongest for fish or fish oil (ARHQ, 2004).

The U.S. Food and Drug Administration (FDA) issued a qualified health claim statement in 2000 that allows EPA/DHA supplements, and in 2004 food products, to print on their labels: "Supportive but not conclusive research shows that consumption of EPA and DHA omega-3 fatty acids may reduce the risk of coronary heart disease." In approving this health claim, the FDA commented:

FRIED FISH IS DETRIMENTAL; BAKED OR BROILED FISH IS PROTECTIVE!

How you prepare fresh fish may affect its heart benefits. Fried fish lose their protective ability, most likely because of destruction or other loss of EPA and DHA.

A ten-year follow-up of more than 84,000 postmenopausal women who participated in the Women's Health Initiative-Observational Study (WHI-OS) compared women who rarely ate broiled or baked fish with women who consumed five or more servings a week (Belin, 2011). The study found that women who consumed five or more servings of broiled or baked fish per week had a 30 percent lower risk of developing heart failure. Conversely, women who had at least one serving a week of fried fish had an almost 50 percent increased risk of incident heart failure, compared with those who rarely ate fried fish. (Additional studies about the effects of fish preparation appear in Chapter 9.)

One advantage of taking EPA and DHA supplements is that you know how much you are getting and that is not affected by cooking.

In particular, the GISSI trial (GISSI, 1999), the clinical trial with the longest duration (3.5 years), the largest sample size (11,324), and that measured both LDL cholesterol and CHD in a diseased population, reported that there were no statistically significant changes in LDL cholesterol, while also reporting a 15 percent decrease in relative risk of coronary heart disease in the diseased population intervention group that consumed omega-3 fatty acids. . . . Thus, in most of the intervention studies, including the GISSI trial, . . . omega-3 fatty acids showed a reduction of risk for coronary heart disease in a

---

2. As we have pointed out, ALA does not offer the same protection against heart disease that is provided by EPA and DHA. ALA is good, but not the same as EPA and DHA. A 2011 study confirmed that there is no association between ALA intake and risk of ischemic heart disease, but a high intake of omega-3 LC-PUFAs had a significant cardioprotective effect (Vedtofte, 2011).

diseased population, but the effect is apparently not working through a mechanism of LDL cholesterol reduction" (Hubbard, 2004).

In the United Kingdom, the National Institute for Health and Clinical Excellence (NICE) issued the following guidance in 2007:

> Patients should be advised to consume at least 7 grams of omega-3 fatty acids per week from two to four portions of oily fish. For patients who have had an MI (heart attack) within three months and who are not achieving 7 grams of omega-3 fatty acids per week, consider providing at least 1 gram daily of omega-3-acid ethyl esters (a form of EPA and DHA) treatment licensed for secondary prevention post MI for up to four years."

Even doses of less than 1 gram a day appear to significantly reduce the risk of fatal coronary heart disease events, but higher amounts offer greater protection. One 2011 study suggests that the lower threshold dose for EPA and DHA combined is 250 mg and above. In the findings of this study, at least 250 mg of EPA and DHA was associated with a 35 percent reduction in the risk of sudden cardiac death and a 17 percent decrease in the risk of total fatal heart attacks (Musa-Veloso, 2011). The researchers pointed out that "prospective observational and intervention data from Japan, where intake of fish is very high, suggest that omega-3 LC-PUFA intakes of 900–1,000 mg per day and greater may confer protection against non-fatal heart attack. Thus, the intake of 250 mg omega-3 LC-PUFAs per day may, indeed, be a minimum target to be achieved by the general population for the promotion of cardiovascular health."

To understand how EPA and DHA produce such dramatic heart benefits, it helps to understand some basics about the heart and vascular system, and how heart disease begins and the processes that can eventually lead to a heart attack.

HOW EPA AND DHA PROTECT AGAINST HEART DISEASE AND HEART ATTACK

Heart disease is really cardiovascular disease, a condition that affects the blood, blood vessels, and heart. There are several types of cardiovascular disease of which CHD, or coronary heart disease, is the most common. In CHD, the myocardium (heart muscle) no longer receives sufficient oxygen for its needs. When there is insufficient oxygen for heart needs, it is called myocardial ischemia or ischemic heart disease (IHD). If the lack of oxygen is severe, the myocardium can't produce energy and the oxygen-starved heart muscle cells die, causing a myocardial infarction (MI), or a heart attack.

The primary cause of CHD is atherosclerosis, which is the result of atheromatous plaque. This plaque consists of lipids, proteins, cell debris, and, yes, cholesterol. The plaque forms in the intima (innermost layer) of the arterial wall and pushes into the lumen (opening), reducing blood flow. The plaques may also fissure, triggering the formation of a blood clot that can lead to a heart attack.

Cardiovascular disease is a multifaceted disease with several risk factors, including, but not necessarily limited to, genetics, lifestyle, and nutrition. The three major categories of risk factors that we will address here are blood clots, arterial narrowing, and heart beat. Figure 8.5 (on the following page) is a diagram showing the three major categories of risk factors that are addressable with dietary corrections. Even if high blood cholesterol is one of the major risk factors for heart disease, dietary cholesterol is only a minor factor for most people, as it does not influence blood cholesterol markedly. It is, however, a major factor for a small minority who have a genetic abnormality (nucleotide polymorphism) called *familial hyperlipidemia* or *hypercholesteremia.* Fish oil does *not* decrease blood cholesterol, despite what many believe. This underlines that there are many risk factors for heart disease other than elevated blood cholesterol. Fish oil or marine omega-3 fatty acids work on these, and as illustrated, they work well!

Each risk category is significant, but of these, blood clotting is the final event in a chain of events leading to a heart attack, and it is also the easiest to alter by nutrients such as EPA and DHA. Although the blood clot in a coronary artery is the final step in a heart attack, we'll begin with it and work our way backward.

Blood Clots

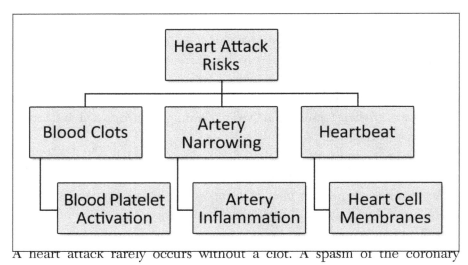

Figure 8.5. The major categories of cardiovascular risks addressable by dietary correction.

artery that shuts off blood flow or causes the heart to fibrillate and be unable to pump blood can result in a heart attack, but the vast majority of heart attacks are caused by a blood clot that forms in a coronary artery that has been constricted by plaque buildup within the artery wall. The majority of strokes are also caused by a blood clot—in this case, a blood clot that forms in a blood vessel that supplies the brain (more on strokes in Chapter 9).

The path to a heart attack is a two-step process. Atherosclerosis, the medical term for narrowed arteries, does not by itself cause heart attacks, but can result in heart pains (angina) due to restriction of the blood flow. (Angina is usually provoked by some sort of physical exertion such as shoveling snow, which increases the heart muscle's demand for oxygen.) Thrombosis (blood clot) and vasoconstriction (constriction and/or spasm of an artery) are the events that usually precipitate a heart attack. The narrowing of an artery begins with an inflammatory response where foam cells (macrophages filled with oxidized LDL) build up under the artery lining. These cells promote the infiltration of various substances through the artery wall into its middle layer. Now the artery can be said to be "diseased" or "dysfunctional" as plaque is formed in the artery interior. As the plaque expands, the wall is pushed into the lumen and the opening where the blood flows through is narrowed. Thus, blood flow is decreased to the heart tissue. The narrowed artery also affects the blood platelets passing by, making the blood sticky and encouraging clot formation at the plaque site.

The key here is that narrowed arteries put the squeeze on blood platelet cells and damage them. Blood platelets are small, disc-shaped, colorless blood cells. They are smaller than red blood cells and there are about 150,000 to 300,000 platelets per microliter (µL) of blood. It is uncanny how much a platelet looks like a chocolate chip cookie when observed through an electron microscope! Even granular proteins on the platelet surface resemble chocolate chips. Furthermore, the buildup of plaque can damage the arterial lining inside, making the platelets "feel" that the lining is a "foreign" surface that they should clump on, as when they stop bleeding.

Platelets play a major role in the process of coagulation of blood to arrest bleeding (homeostasis). When bleeding begins, the vessel constricts, a protein called *tissue factor* is released, and a protein (collagen) in the vessel wall is exposed. When tissue factor is released by the blood vessel wall, a lipoprotein on the surface of the platelet called *platelet factor 3* is activated and reacts with blood factors to promote the formation of a platelet plug and initiate other steps in the blood-clotting mechanism. When platelet factor 3 is activated, the platelet changes shape and is said to be activated.

Platelets, however, can be activated even when there is no bleeding, and this is not good. If they are activated, they still tend to aggregate or clump together and initiate an undesirable blood clot, which can block blood flow through the vessel and result in a heart attack or stroke. If this undesirable blood clot is stationary, it is called a thrombus, and if it travels through the vessel, it is called an embolism. An embolism can reach a narrower vessel and become a thrombus. Platelets can also be activated by smoking, stress, diabetes, and certain nutritional deficiencies. In addition, as people age, a greater percentage of their platelets tend to be undesirably activated.

A critical factor in preventing a heart attack then is to maintain the proper slipperiness of blood cells and prevent a blood clot from forming in the coronary arteries. As Dr. Dyerberg found during his expeditions and as we have discussed in earlier chapters, EPA reduces the tendency of blood to clot and increases the slipperiness of blood. EPA regulates the blood's own clotting system such that the clotting tendency is lowered. EPA is converted to anti-inflammatory eicosanoids that tune the clotting system toward a lower level of activity than when eicosanoids are only formed from pro-inflammatory arachidonic acid (AA). The shift is rather modest, and does not give rise to concern regarding bleeding risk at 1–4 grams, the dosage typically recommended for general nutritional purposes and with special medical conditions.

Now we understand even more about how both EPA and DHA affect platelet aggregation. Platelet "microparticles" are a reliable marker of platelet hyperactivity and platelet aggregation. A single dose of EPA or DHA can decrease the activity of platelet microparticles by 20 percent. A study conducted at the University of Newcastle in New South Wales, Australia, led by Dr. M. L. Garg, concluded, "This study demonstrates that a single dose of EPA-rich oil significantly inhibits platelet micropar- ticle activity in parallel with a reduction in platelet aggregation, while supplementation with DHA-rich oils reduces platelet aggregation *inde- pendent* of microparticle activity" (Phang, 2011). The total amount of EPA and DHA was 1 gram (1,000 mg) in each group, with the EPA-rich group receiving a single dose of 0.833 mg of EPA plus 0.167 mg DHA, while the DHA-rich group received a single dose of 0.167 mg EPA plus 0.833 mg DHA.

Furthermore, EPA and DHA decrease levels of thromboxane A2. This pro-inflammatory eicosanoid produced by activated blood platelets also induces vasoconstriction (narrowing of blood vessels), thereby reducing blood flow and increasing blood pressure. Prostaglandin I2 (also called prostacyclin I2 or PGI2) inhibits platelet activation. A diet rich in EPA and DHA lowers the cell membrane AA content (via competition) and thus reduces the levels of AA-derived eicosanoids thromboxane A2. At the same time, an EPA/DHA-rich diet promotes the formation of throm- boxane A3 and prostaglandin I3, which keep blood platelets slippery and free flowing.

Table 8.2 summarizes the primary way in which EPA and DHA protect against heart attacks. By helping reduce the clumping together of platelets, EPA and DHA reduce the risk of a potentially fatal blood clot forming in a coronary artery.

TABLE 8.2. PRIMARY CARDIOPROTECTIVE ACTION OF EPA AND DHA	
1	
Risk	Blood clots in the coronary arteries that shut off blood flow and cause a heart attack
What EPA and DHA do to reduce risk	Form compounds that reduce clotting
How	Form anti-thrombotic eicosanoids, including thromboxane A3 and prostaglandin I3
Result	Most effective dietary intervention known

Artery Narrowing

Chronic inflammation is now recognized as the major underlying cause of heart disease. This shift in medical thinking away from the cholesterol theory is illustrated by a seminal report in the AHA journal *Circulation* in 2002 (Libby, 2002).

To quote from the article's abstract,

Atherosclerosis, formerly considered a bland lipid storage disease, actually involves an ongoing inflammatory response. Recent advances in basic science have established a fundamental role for inflammation in mediating all stages of this disease from initiation through progression and, ultimately, the thrombotic complications of atherosclerosis. These new findings provide important links between risk factors and the mechanisms of atherogenesis [the process of plaque formation in the inner lining of the arteries]. Clinical studies have shown that this emerging biology of inflammation in atherosclerosis applies directly to human patients.

The abstract continues,

Moreover, certain treatments that reduce coronary risk also limit inflammation. In the case of lipid lowering with statins (popular heart drugs), this anti-inflammatory effect does not appear to correlate with reduction in low-density lipoprotein levels.

Well, EPA and DHA have considerable anti-inflammatory actions! In 2009 the journal published an update that concluded,

> Multiple independent pathways of evidence now pinpoint inflammation as a key regulatory process that links multiple risk factors for atherosclerosis and its complications with altered arterial biology. This revolution in our thinking about the pathophysiology of atherosclerosis has begun to provide clinical insight and practical tools that may aid patient management.

As explained in Chapter 4, vascular inflammation can lead to lipid deposits in the walls of arteries. EPA and DHA help prevent formation of these deposits. By way of a mechanism parallel to that used to control blood clotting, EPA and DHA attenuate the body's inflammatory reaction. This is due to the formation of eicosanoids but also to substances known as resolvins, maresins, and protectins that are made from both EPA and DHA. These compounds block the migration of white blood cells across the walls of small blood vessels—a crucial step in causing inflammation (Tull, 2009). They also promote resolution of the inflammatory process in the body. For example, people with arthritis experience pain relief when taking fish oil supplements due to attenuation of the inflammatory process. In the same way, omega-3 fatty acids attenuate the inflammatory process in the vessel walls and thereby the progression of the atherosclerotic process. These substances are only formed by EPA and DHA and not from AA, which once again underscores our need for a proper intake of EPA and DHA.

An indication of omega-3 fatty acids' beneficial effect on inflammation is that people with a high omega-3 intake have lower C-reactive protein (CRP) levels in their blood as compared to people with a low omega-3 intake. CRP rises during inflammatory processes in the body and is a marker of the degree and extent of the inflammation. People with elevated levels of CRP are at an increased risk for ischemic heart disease. This is true even for apparently healthy men and women who have normal cholesterol levels. Tests of CRP levels are now routinely used to assess the risk of heart disease; low risk is associated with CRP levels of 1 mg per liter (mg/L) or less, high risk with levels greater than 3 mg/L. By lowering inflammatory activity in the body, supplementation with fish oil adds an extra-protective facet to the broad spectrum of beneficial effects of omega-3 LC-PUFAs on ischemic heart disease.

Now we can add a second function to the table of heart disease causes and how EPA and DHA reduce these risks. See Table 8.3.

TABLE 8.3. TWO CARDIOPROTECTIVE ACTIONS OF EPA AND DHA		
	1	**2**
Risk	Blood clots in the coronary arteries that shut off blood flow and cause a heart attack	Artery narrowing and deposits
What EPA and DHA do to reduce risk	Form compounds that reduce clotting	Control the inflammation process and prevent formation of deposits
How	Form anti-thrombotic eicosanoids, including thromboxane A3 and prostaglandin I3	Produce anti-inflammatory eicosanoids and docosanoids such as leukotriene A5, protectins, resolvins, and maresins
Result	Most effective dietary intervention known	Highly effective dietary intervention

The term "hardening of the arteries" is often used to describe arteries that not only have plaque (deposits), but also are calcified and stiffened. In addition to reducing the risk of arterial deposits, EPA and DHA also work to keep the arteries properly elastic and flexible. Remember the saying "You are as old as your arteries"? This refers to the elasticity and flexibility of your arteries.

An Australian review of the scientific literature supports the science behind EPA and DHA reducing arterial stiffness (Pase, 2011). The study states that "supplementation with omega-3 fatty acids offers a scientifically supported means of reducing arterial stiffness. Reduction in arterial stiffness by omega-3 fatty acids may account for some of their purported cardioprotective effects."

Triglycerides

Among the blood lipids historically associated with narrowing of the arteries and the development of atherosclerosis, most attention had been paid to cholesterol. Omega-3 fatty acids have no effect on blood cholesterol, but they do on other blood lipids that play a role in atherosclerosis. One of these is blood triglycerides. Blood triglycerides can be elevated by many factors, which include high alcohol intake, being overweight, and having diabetes mellitus.

Historically, the association between elevated triglycerides in the blood and cardiovascular disease has been of strong interest to physicians. We discussed triglycerides in Chapter 2, pointing out that this is how fatty acids are normally stored and transported, whether the fats be in foods, adipose tissue, or the blood. Having elevated triglycerides in the blood indicates that higher than normal amounts of fats are being carried. For reasons not yet known, there is an association of elevated blood triglycerides and heart disease. Thus, physicians like to normalize this risk factor.

Large epidemiological studies suggest that an increased non-fasting blood triglyceride level increases ischemic heart disease risk many fold (Nordestgaard, 2007). Other studies have further shown that for each 10 mg per deciliter (mg/dL) decrement in triglyceride level, the incidence of death and heart attack was lowered by 1.6 percent (Bansal, 2007).

EPA and DHA have profound triglyceride-lowering effects, comparable to that of lipid-lowering drugs, but without their side effects! It is well known that fish oil—in appropriately high amounts (2–4 grams per day)—normalizes blood triglyceride levels. EPA and DHA lower triglyceride formation in the liver and also decrease the release of very-low-density lipoprotein (VLDL) into the blood. The AHA recommends 3 grams of EPA and DHA daily to normalize blood triglycerides. Interestingly, this is a higher intake than recommended for the prevention of other aspects of cardiovascular disease, which is 1 gram.

EPA and DHA separately have each been shown to lower blood triglyceride levels (Bernstein, 2011). Table 8.4 lists a third major way in which EFA and DHA protect against heart attacks and heart disease.

TABLE 8.4. THREE CARDIOPROTECTIVE ACTIONS OF EPA/DHA

	1	2	3
Risk	Blood clots in the coronary arteries that shut off blood flow and cause a heart attack	Artery narrowing and deposits	Elevated blood triglycerides
What EPA and DHA do to reduce risk	Form compounds that reduce clotting	Control the inflammation process and prevent formation of deposits	Normalize blood triglyceride levels
How	Form anti-thrombotic eicosanoids, including thromboxane A3 and prostaglandin I3	Produce anti-inflammatory eicosanoids and docosanoids such as leukotriene A5, protectins, resolvins, and maresins	Mechanism not known
Result	Most effective dietary intervention known	Highly effective dietary intervention	Reduction of a popular risk factor

The consumption of omega-3 fatty acids leads to a 10–33 percent decrease of triglyceride levels. The effect is dose-dependent; meaning that the higher the intake of EPA and DHA, the greater the decrease across all different populations (including healthy people, people with dyslipidemia, diabetes, or known cardiovascular risk factors), especially in those having very high triglyceride levels to begin with.

Heart Beat

The average human heart, beating at 72 beats per minute, will beat approximately 3 billion times during an eighty-year lifespan. Most people seldom think about the tireless beating of their heart. That is, until they feel a *palpitation,* which is an abnormal beat known as a premature ventricular contraction (PVC). *Arrhythmias* are abnormalities of the heart rate and rhythm caused by improper functioning of electrical system cells in the heart.

There are different kinds of arrhythmias. Palpitations are the most common and refer to the feeling of a pounding heartbeat, whether regular or irregular. *Tachycardia* is an abnormal increase in resting heart rate to more than 100 beats per minute. A *fibrillation* is an irregular heartbeat that may be episodic or chronic and is characterized by a very rapid heartbeat, in which the four chambers in the heart (two atria and two ventricles) flutter rather than beat. Heart arrhythmias interfere with the heart's ability to efficiently deliver blood to the body. In some cases, heart arrhythmias can be a sign of underlying heart disease. Other arrhythmias, such as ventricular tachycardia and ventricular fibrillation, are more significant because they cause the heart to beat very fast and can be life-threatening.

Regular beating of the heart, which is a striated muscle, is achieved as a result of the inherent (intrinsic) rhythmicity of cardiac cells. No nerves are located within the heart itself, and no outside regulatory mechanisms are necessary to stimulate the muscle to contract rhythmically. Each cardiac cell has its own intrinsic contraction rhythm, which is dependent on the presence and proper ratio of calcium, sodium, and potassium ions in order to maintain a regular heart rhythm.

The fluidity of cell membranes is critical for optimal functioning of the calcium channels, and, as we know, EPA and DHA are critical for maintaining membrane fluidity. Dr. A. Leaf, a professor of clinical medicine at Harvard Medical School, has found in his studies of individual heart cells that omega-3 fatty acids block excessive sodium and calcium currents in the heart, which are associated with dangerous changes in heart rhythm. Scientists now believe that fish oils act by taking up residence in the membranes of heart cells and alter the cells' electrical properties, making it harder for dangerous spasms to start. "If you have a heart attack—heaven forbid—[hopefully] the fatty acids are already in the heart . . . and prevent arrhythmia," observes the researcher (Leaf, 1988).

Numerous studies have found EPA and DHA help normalize and prevent atrial and ventricular arrhythmias. Let's look briefly at a few.

Atrial Arrhythmias

Atrial fibrillation is a type of arrhythmia that is caused by erratic electrical signals originating from the atria. It is the most common irregular heart rhythm that starts in the atria.

In 2009 a Finnish study of omega-3 LC-PUFAs and atrial fibrillation found support for the nutrients' protective effect. A total of 2,174 men from the Kuopio Ischemic Heart Disease Risk Factor Study, ages forty-two to sixty and free of atrial fibrillation at enrollment in 1984 to 1989, were studied. EPA, DHA, and docosapentaenoic acid (DPA, an omega-3 fatty acid) levels were measured in each of the participants at the time of their enrollment. During the average follow-up time of seventeen and a half years, 240 atrial fibrillation events occurred. When researchers reevaluated the fatty acid measurements, they found that men in the highest quartile of concentrations (>5.33 percent) had a reduced risk of developing atrial fibrillation when compared to men in the lowest quartile (<3.61 percent). When each fatty acid was evaluated individually, only DHA was associated with the risk of developing atrial fibrillation; again men in the top 25 percent with more DHA were at less risk than men in the bottom 25 percent with less DHA. The researchers concluded, "An increased concentration of long-chain ω-3 [omega-3] PUFAs in serum may protect against atrial fibrillation. Serum docosahexaenoic acid concentration had the greatest impact" (Virtanen, 2009).

Atrial fibrillation is a common complication after coronary-artery bypass grafting (CABG) operations. The surgery is routinely done when three major arteries are diseased, and as with any surgical procedure. It involves some risk; nationwide, about 1–3 percent of bypass patients do not survive the operation or recovery period. Experimental data have shown anti-arrhythmic effects of EPA and DHA on heart cells, causing researchers to assess the efficacy of LC-PUFAs for the prevention of atrial fibrillation after CABG. In one study, fifty-two patients were randomly assigned to the interventional group, while fifty served as controls. The control group was given free fatty acids from soy. The interventional group was given fish oil at a dosage of 100 mg of fish oil per kilogram (kg) of body weight per day. The primary endpoint was the postoperative development of atrial fibrillation, as assessed by surface electrocardiogram (ECG); the secondary endpoint was the length of stay in the intensive care unit (ICU). The demographic, clinical, and surgical characteristics of the patients in the two groups were similar. Postoperative atrial fibrillation occurred in fifteen patients (30.6 percent) in the control and in nine (17.3 percent) in the fish oil group. After CABG surgery, the fish oil group had to be treated in the ICU for a shorter time than the control patients. No adverse effects were observed. The researchers concluded that pre-operative fish oil reduces the incidence of atrial fibrillation after surgery and leads to a shorter stay in the ICU and in hospital (Heidt, 2009).

The issue of atrial fibrillation and fish oil has met some controversy, in that some negative studies have been reported. Recently, however, it was found that chronic fish oil ingestion in humans attenuates atrial tachycardia that manifests after reversion of persistent atrial arrhythmias to normal rhythm. This suggests that fish oils may target or even reverse underlying cellular and/or structural damage that occurs in response to persistent atrial arrhythmias (Kumar, 2012). Another study concluded, "Omega-3 LC-PUFA supplementation commenced more than one month prior to electrical cardioversion [the process of restarting the heart with an electric shock] and continued thereafter reduces the recurrence of persistent atrial fibrillation" (Kumar, 2011).

Any lingering doubt about the positive effect of omega-3 LC-PUFAs on atrial fibrillation should vanish with the publication of the Cardiovascular Heart Study by a research team at the Harvard School of Public Health in a 2012 issue of the journal *Circulation*. The study examined circulating levels of omega-3 LC PUFAs, rather than relying merely on dietary intake. The study found those in the top 25 percent of omega-3 LC-PUFA levels had a 29 percent reduction in risk of atrial fibrillation compared to those in the lowest 25 percent levels. The researchers reported, "Our findings suggest that omega-3 (LC) fatty acids could be beneficial for the prevention of onset of atrial fibrillation in older individuals, a group at particularly high risk."

Interestingly, the risk reduction is more strongly associated with DHA than EPA. In this prospective study, data from 3,326 men and women with an average age of seventy-four were analyzed for fourteen years from 1992 to 2006. Over the course of the study, 789 cases of atrial fibrillation were reported. A finding of the study was that the highest average levels of both total omega-3 LC-PUFAs and DHA were associated with an atrial fibrillation risk reduction of about 25 percent. Each 1 percent higher of total omega-3 LC PUFAs was associated with a 9 percent lower risk of atrial fibrillation. However, the individual omega-3 LC-PUFAs EPA and DPA were associated with lower atrial fibrillation risk (Wu, 2012).

When comparing levels of DHA alone (rather than total omega-3 LC

PUFAs), those in the top 25 percent of DHA blood levels had a 23 percent reduction. Thus, DHA alone and total omega-3 LC PUFAs were found to have a direct inverse relationship to atrial fibrillation, whereas EPA and DPA individually were not found to have an association.

Ventricular Arrhythmias

In 2005 Dr. Leaf and his colleagues extended their fish oil and fibrillation research to patients having implanted cardioverter defibrillators (ICD, an electronic device that constantly monitors heart rhythm). When the ICD detects a very fast, abnormal heart rhythm, it delivers energy to the heart muscle, which causes the heart to beat in a normal rhythm again. They found that fish oil appears to reduce potentially fatal ventricular arrhythmias in patients with ICDs.

In the 2005 study, 402 patients with ICDs were randomly assigned to double-blind treatment with either a fish oil or an olive oil daily supplement for twelve months. Patients who received treatment with the fish oil supplement tended to have a longer time before the first event (either from ventricular tachycardia or ventricular fibrillation) or of death from any cause (showing risk reduction of 28 percent). When therapies for probable episodes of ventricular tachycardia or ventricular fibrillation were included, the risk reduction became significant at 31 percent. For those who stayed on the protocol for at least eleven months, the anti-arrhythmic benefit of fish oil was improved for those with confirmed events (risk reduction of 38 percent). "This study provides evidence," the researchers concluded, "that for individuals at high risk of fatal ventricular arrhythmias, regular daily ingestion of fish oil fatty acids may significantly reduce potentially fatal ventricular arrhythmias" (Leaf, 2005). However, also studies not finding such an effect have been published, so we are, as in many fields of medicine, in the process of gaining clear knowledge.

It has been suggested that 2–4 grams per day of total LC-PUFA would be useful in reducing ventricular arrhythmias. Animal studies with induced ventricular arrhythmias show that EPA and DHA markedly decrease the arrhythmias. An anti-arrhythmia effect is observed when the DHA content of membranes exceeds 20 percent.

Table 8.5 lists the four major ways in which EPA and DHA reduce the risk of heart disease and heart attacks.

TABLE 8.5. FOUR MAJOR CARDIOPROTECTIVE ACTIONS OF EPA/DHA				
	1	2	3	4
Risk	Blood clots in the coronary arteries that shut off blood flow and cause a heart attack	Artery narrowing and deposits	Elevated blood triglycerides	Inefficient heartbeat
What EPA and DHA do to reduce risk	Form compounds that reduce clotting	Control the inflammation process and prevent formation of deposits	Normalize blood triglyceride levels	Normalize the cell membranes of the heart
How	Form anti-thrombotic eicosanoids, including thromboxane A3 and prostaglandin I3	Produce anti-inflammatory eicosanoids and docosanoids such as leukotriene A5, protectins, resolvins, and maresins	Mechanism not known	Form the proper phospholipids and promote cell membrane fluidity
Result	Most effective dietary intervention known	Highly effective dietary intervention	Reduction of a popular risk factor	Normalization of heart rhythm

We have not included lowering blood pressure in the tables of major effects of EPA and DHA in lowering risk of heart disease, but they do exert a minor influence. Recent evidence suggests that at least a part of the protective effect of EPA and DHA is mediated by a relatively small but significant decrease in blood pressure level. In fact, omega-3 LC-PU-FAs exhibit wide-ranging biological actions that include regulating both quality of vascular tone and function, and sodium levels, partly competing with omega-6 PUFAs for common metabolic enzymes, and thereby decreasing the production of vasoconstrictor rather than vasodilator and anti-inflammatory eicosanoids. The final results are improved dilation and "smoothness" of both small and large arteries. Clinical trials involving normotensive and hypertensive patients, diabetics, and elderly subjects confirm this. Meta-analyses show that omega-3 LC-PUFAs are able to slightly, but significantly, reduce high blood pressure (Cicero, 2009; Liu, 2011).

The AHA, among other major medical organizations, now acknowledges the research showing that EPA and DHA decrease the risk of heart attacks **caused by blood clots**, decrease arrhythmias, decrease inflammation and triglyceride levels, and slightly lower blood pressure. We agree! To read more, a bibliography of EPA and DHA and heart disease can be found online at www.omega-research.com/research11.php ?catid=8&-subcat=73.

In the next chapter we will take a brief look at the role of omega-3 LC-PUFAs in reducing the risk of stroke.

9

Stroke

A stroke is a cerebrovascular accident that is caused by an interruption of blood flow within the brain. This interruption can be caused by a blockage from a blood clot that originates in the brain or migrates there from elsewhere in the body, or by a hemorrhage from a weak vessel that ruptures in the brain and leaks blood. If the blood supply to the brain cells is interrupted for longer than a few minutes, the cells do not get the oxygen they need and die. As a result, the affected area of the brain is unable to function, and depending on what it is responsible for, the body is impaired.

Prevention of stroke is a major issue in modern medicine. In the United States, stroke affects more than 700,000 people and claims more than 160,000 lives each year, whereas 4.8 million patients suffer from continuing complications from strokes in previous years. In addition, the cost of treatment for stroke reached $53.6 billion in 2004. In comparison to cardiac events, stroke has a higher tendency to leave temporary and/or permanent disabilities, requires long-term rehabilitation and care, and is thus associated with key problems such as increased family burden and medical costs. Although the predominant risk factor for stroke is high blood pressure, other risk factors exist such as diabetes, atherosclerosis, smoking, atrial fibrillation, and heavy consumption of alcohol.

HOW EPA AND DHA WORK TO PROTECT AGAINST STROKE

There are two major types of stroke: ischemic stroke and hemorrhagic stroke. Approximately 87 percent of strokes are ischemic strokes. They occur when a blood vessel that supplies blood to the brain is blocked by a blood clot, causing severely reduced blood flow (ischemia). This may happen in two ways: A clot may form in an artery that is already very narrow; this is called a *thrombotic stroke.* Or a clot may break off from another place in the blood vessels of the brain, or from some other part of the body, and travel up to the brain and become lodged in a narrower artery; this is called *cerebral embolism,* or an *embolic stroke.*

Hemorrhagic strokes account for the remaining 13 percent of strokes. They occur when a blood vessel in part of the brain becomes weak and bursts open, causing blood to leak (hemorrhage) into the brain. Some people have defects in the blood vessels of the brain that makes this more likely. Bleeding within the brain is called *intracerebral hemorrhage;* bleeding in the membrane surrounding the brain is called *subarachnoid hemorrhage.*

Keep Arteries Healthy and Free of Clots

Ischemic strokes may be caused by clogged arteries. Another common cause is fibrillation of the atria (upper chambers) of the heart. When the atria dilate and fibrillate, they cause the heart to beat fast and irregularly. Small blood clots have a tendency to form, and these clots can then travel by arterial blood and land in the brain causing a stroke. (Due to this risk, people with atrial fibrillation are often advised by their physicians to be on anticoagulation medication and take fish oil!) In Chapter 8, we discussed the role of EPA and DHA in reducing blood clots that can cause heart attacks and also how EPA and DHA reduce atrial fibrillation. The omega-3, long-chain polyunsaturated fatty acids (LC-PUFAs) EPA and DHA reduce platelet adhesion (stickiness), thereby reducing the tendency for blood to clot. They also reduce inflammation in the artery walls that leads to the build-up of plaque that narrows the arteries. Both actions help maintain healthy arteries free of clots, including in the cerebral arteries in the brain.

Hemorrhagic strokes can be due to defects in the blood vessels of the brain, but high blood pressure is most often the leading cause of such artery rupture. In fact, high blood pressure is associated with a 35–50 percent risk of all strokes—ischemic and hemorrhagic. Just as the pressure in a power washer can burst a garden hose but not a high-pressure hose, high blood pressure physically damages arteries and can create weak places that rupture easily, or thin spots that fill up with blood and balloon out from the artery wall.

It is natural to wonder whether the reduction in platelet adhesion and blood clotting is a concern regarding strokes due to internal bleeding in the brain. The Eskimos, with their 14 grams of EPA and DHA per day, did experience an increase in stroke incidence because their relative amount of hemorrhagic stroke was increased. However, this was compensated by the far lower death rates from heart attacks and lower thrombotic strokes. The amounts of EPA and DHA that we recommend (1 gram per day for preventive measures; up to 4 grams per day for treatment of some conditions) have not shown any increase in risk of bleeding within the brain, nor elsewhere.

Lower Triglyceride Levels

Another suggested mechanism that explains how EPA and DHA reduce stroke risk is their effectiveness at lowering both fasting and non-fasting blood triglyceride levels. As you may also recall from Chapter 8, studies have found that dosages of 2–4 grams of EPA and DHA a day can substantially reduce both fasting and non-fasting blood triglyceride levels (Skulas-Ray, 2011). One such study, a placebo-controlled, double-blind, randomized, three-period crossover trial (eight weeks of treatment, followed by six weeks without treatment), compared the effects of 0.85–4 grams of EPA and DHA a day in twenty-three men and three postmenopausal women with moderately high triglyceride levels. The higher dose of EPA and DHA lowered triglycerides by 27 percent compared with the placebo (Kris-Etherton, 2011).

In the Copenhagen City Heart Study, a prospective Danish epidemiological cohort study, triglyceride levels were collected from 13,956 men and women, ages twenty through ninety-three, in 1976 and then followed for up to thirty-three years. It was found that high non-fasting triglyceride levels were associated with substantial increased risk of ischemic stroke. Men with the highest non-fasting triglyceride level had a 2.5 times higher stroke risk versus men with the lowest non-fasting levels. Corresponding values for women were 3.8 times higher stroke risk (Freiberg, 2008).

Help Stabilize Plaque

Supporting evidence for the protective role of fish comes from carotid artery (neck artery) ultrasound studies, which have demonstrated that less carotid plaque is present in those with the greatest intake of omega-3 fatty acids from fish (Hino, 2004).

One study found that fish oil had positive effects on the structure of carotid plaque. In this clinical trial, 162 people who had severe carotid plaque and were scheduled for carotid endarterectomy (surgical removal of the plaque) were randomly given fish oil, sunflower oil, or no treatment, while waiting for their procedures. (The median waiting time was forty-two days.) Once the plaque was removed surgically, it was examined microscopically. Participants who took the fish oil had less inflammation in their plaque and thicker tissue covering its fatty core: two markers of more stable plaque. Those taking the sunflower oil or receiving no treatment had unstable plaque with greater inflammation and thinner, less sturdy covering tissue. This suggests that consuming fish oil for just less than two months substantially stabilizes carotid plaque, making it less likely to rupture and fragment, and thus cause a stroke. The researchers reported that "Atherosclerotic plaques readily incorporate ω-3 [omega-3] PUFAs from fish oil supplementation, inducing changes that can enhance stability of atherosclerotic plaques. By contrast, increased consumption of omega-6 PUFAs does not affect carotid plaque fatty-acid composition or stability over the time course studied here. Stability of plaques could explain [previously observed] reductions in non-fatal and fatal cardiovascular events associated with increased omega-3 PUFA intake" (Thies, 2003). A similar study found that a low serum EPA level and a low EPA/AA ratio were associated with high vulnerability of atherosclerotic plaques (Kashiyama, 2011).

INFLUENTIAL STUDIES OF STROKE EFFECTS

Long-term clinical studies for stroke prevention are expensive and difficult to design, so most of the evidence we have thus far comes from population-based studies. Several studies suggest a strong relationship between fish intake and reduced stroke risk (Iso, 2001; He, 2001, 2002). Let's take a look at how some of the body of science has developed.

Fish Intake and Stroke Incidence

In 2001 Harvard researchers published their study data of a cohort from the Nurses' Health Study in the *Journal of the American Medical Association* in which they found that "higher consumption of fish and omega-3 polyunsaturated fatty acids is associated with a reduced risk of thrombotic infarction (stroke by blood clot blockage), primarily among women who do not take aspirin regularly, but is not related to risk of hemorrhagic stroke" (Iso, 2001).

The Harvard researchers studied a cohort of women in the Nurses' Health Study, ages thirty-four to fifty-nine, who were free from prior diagnosed cardiovascular disease and elevated cholesterol levels and who had completed a food-frequency questionnaire at the beginning of the study in 1980 that provided information on their consumption of fish and other frequently eaten foods. The 79,839 women were followed up for fourteen years.

After 1,086,261 person-years of follow-up, 574 incidents of stroke were documented. Of these, there were 303 thrombotic strokes, 119 subarachnoid hemorrhages, 62 intracerebral hemorrhages, and 90 strokes of undetermined type. Compared with women who ate fish less than once per month, those with a higher intake of fish had a lower risk of stroke. Women who consumed fish one to three times per month experienced 7 percent fewer strokes; one time per week, 22 percent fewer strokes; two to four times per week, 27 percent fewer strokes; and five or more times per week, 52 percent fewer strokes.

Among certain types of stroke, a significantly reduced risk of thrombotic stroke was found among women who ate fish two or more times per week (51 percent reduction). Women whose intake of LC-PUFAs was in the highest 20 percent of participants reduced their risk of total stroke and thrombotic stroke, by 28 percent and 33 percent, respectively. When divided into groups by aspirin use, and fish and omega-3 LC-PUFA intakes were inversely associated with risk of thrombotic stroke, primarily among women who did not regularly take aspirin. (Aspirin reduces clotting tendency by inhibiting thromboxane production by interfering with enzymes called cyclooxygenase-2, or COX-2. Aspirin has an anti-platelet effect by inhibiting the production of thromboxane, which under normal circumstances binds platelet molecules together to create a patch over damaged walls of blood vessels.) There was no association between fish or omega-3 LC-PUFA intake and risk of hemorrhagic stroke.

In 2002, in the same medical journal, the Harvard researchers published a study on stroke in men. They concluded, "Our findings suggest that eating fish once per month or more can reduce the risk of ischemic stroke in men." The Harvard researchers used the data from the Health Professionals Follow-up Study, a U.S. prospective cohort study with twelve years of follow-up. The study included a total of 43,671 men, ages forty to seventy-five, who completed a detailed food-frequency questionnaire and who were free of cardiovascular disease at baseline in 1986. The researchers documented 608 strokes during the twelve-year follow-up period, including 377 ischemic, 106 hemorrhagic, and 125 unclassified strokes. Compared with men who consumed fish less than once per month, the risk of ischemic stroke was 43 percent lower among those who ate fish one to three times per month. However, a higher frequency of fish intake was not associated with appreciable further risk reduction; the risk of ischemic stroke was 46 percent lower for men who consumed fish five or more times per week. The inverse association between fish intake and risk of ischemic stroke was not materially modified by use of aspirin. No significant associations were found between fish or omega-3 LC-PUFA intake and risk of hemorrhagic stroke (He, 2002).

In 2004 Northwestern University researchers did a meta-analysis of selected studies. They identified nine independent cohorts from eight different studies and found that compared with those who never consumed fish or who ate fish less than once per month, the risk of ischemic stroke was 9 percent lower for individuals eating fish one to three times per month; 13 percent lower for individuals eating fish once per week;

18 percent lower for individuals eating fish two to four times per week; and 31 percent lower for individuals eating fish five or more times per week. "These results suggest," the researchers wrote, "that intake of fish is inversely related to risk of stroke, particularly ischemic stroke. Fish consumption as seldom as one to three times per month may protect against the incidence of ischemic stroke" (He, 2004).

A review of prospective studies regarding the association between fish consumption and stroke risk was undertaken by Drs. S. C. Larsson and N. Orsini of the National Institute of Environmental Medicine at the Karolinska Institute in Stockholm. Their meta-analysis involved fifteen selected prospective studies that totaled 9,360 stroke events among 383,838 participants. They determined that an increment of three servings per week in fish consumption was associated with a 6 percent reduction in risk of total stroke. Nine of the fifteen studies reported results for the two stroke types. The results were the same—a 10 percent reduction in risk for both ischemic stroke and hemorrhagic stroke (Larsson, 2011).

To benefit from these protective effects of EPA and DHA in fish, studies show that the method of cooking the fish matters. To learn more, see the inset below.

ALL FORMS OF PREPARING FISH ARE NOT EQUAL

It is the fatty, cold-water fish such as mackerel, cod, salmon, herring, sardines, and tuna that are especially rich in EPA and DHA. However, the method of cooking the fish is also critical. In Chapter 8 on heart disease, we briefly mentioned that all forms of preparing fish are not equal. Broiled and baked fish are protective, whereas fried fish are detrimental for heart health. Well, the same findings hold true for stroke! By 2005 it was becoming clear that *fried* fish was not protective. A study published in the *Archives of Internal Medicine* stated, "Among elderly individuals, consumption of tuna or other broiled or baked fish is associated with lower risk of ischemic stroke, while intake of fried fish or fish sandwiches is associated with higher risk. These results suggest that fish consumption may influence stroke risk late in life" (Mozaffarian, 2005).

Inhabitants of the Stroke Belt—an area of the American South made up of North Carolina, South Carolina, Georgia, Alabama, Mississippi, Louisiana, Tennessee, and Arkansas—are 20 percent more likely to die from stroke than those living in the rest of the country. And those in the Stroke Buckle, an area of the Stroke

Belt that includes the coastal plains of North Carolina, South Carolina, and Georgia, are 40 percent more likely to die from stroke.

In a study published in *Neurology*, researchers examined data on 21,675 people participating in a study program called REGARDS, for Reasons for Geographic and Racial Differences in Stroke. The study found that along with a higher consumption of fried fish, people living in the Stroke Belt are less likely to have an adequate intake of non-fried fish (defined in the study as two or more servings of non-fried fish per week based on guidelines from the American Heart Association). "These differences in fish consumption may be one of the potential reasons for the racial and geographic differences in stroke incidence and mortality," says Dr. F. Nahab of Emory University in Atlanta and lead author of the study.

It also found that African-Americans are more likely to eat two or more servings of fried fish per week than whites. A serving is considered 3 ounces of fish (Nahab, 2011).

Fish Oil Supplements and Stroke Incidence

In 2008 the effects of EPA on stroke incidence were investigated as part of a large Japanese trial known as the Japan EPA Lipid Intervention Study (JELIS). The primary purpose of the five-year JELIS trial was to examine the preventive effect of EPA against coronary heart disease in more than 18,000 patients with high cholesterol. One group (9,319) of study participants received statins only, and the other group (9,326) statins with 1,800 milligrams (mg) of EPA per day. After a follow-up of nearly 4.6 years, the EPA was shown to have significantly suppressed the incidence of cardiovascular events such as stroke, fatal or non-fatal heart attacks, and coronary artery bypass surgery.

Researchers then conducted a sub-analysis to investigate the ability of EPA to prevent an occurrence (primary prevention) and reoccurrence (secondary prevention) of stroke in those in the JELIS trial without and with a prior history of stroke. Primary prevention of stroke occurred in 114 (1.3 percent) of 8,862 in the no-EPA group and in 133 (1.5 percent) of 8,841 in the EPA group. No statistically significant difference in total stroke incidence in those people studied with high blood cholesterol and treated with statin drugs without a history of stroke was observed between the no-EPA and the EPA groups. In the secondary prevention

subgroup—people with a recurring history of stroke with high blood cholesterol and being treated with statin drugs—stroke occurred in 48 (10.5
percent) of 457 in the no-EPA group and in 33 (6.8 percent) of 485 in
the EPA group, showing a 20 percent reduction in recurrent stroke in the
EPA group. This demonstrated that EPA had a significant and important
effect on stroke recurrence, particularly of ischemic stroke, in people
with a history of strokes. The researchers concluded, "Administration of
highly purified EPA appeared to reduce the risk of recurrent stroke in a
Japanese population of hypercholesterolemic patients receiving low-dose
statin therapy" (Tanaka, 2008).

Predictor of Stroke Risk

In the preceding chapter, we looked at a new method of assessing risks
of cardiovascular disease that is more accurate than existing blood risk
factors such as elevated cholesterol or triglycerides. This new test, called
the omega-3 index, determines the ratio of EPA and DHA to the total
fatty acid content of red blood cells. A South Korean research group
has applied this concept to stroke. In 2009 they reported their findings
in *Nutrition Research.*

The case-control study recruited 120 subjects, with forty cases each
of hemorrhagic stroke, ischemic stroke, and unaffected controls. Patients
with a family history of hemorrhagic stroke had a significantly increased
risk for that. The omega-3 index was negatively associated with the risk of
both hemorrhagic and ischemic strokes. The study also tested other fatty
acids for their effect on stroke risk. Saturated fatty acids were positively
associated, whereas omega-6 linoleic acid (LA) and omega-3 alpha-linolenic acid (ALA) were negatively associated with risk of ischemic stroke.
Monounsaturated omega-9 oleic acid increased the odds of hemorrhagic
stroke. EPA and DHA were significantly lower in patients with both subtypes of hemorrhagic stroke: subarachnoid hemorrhage and intracerebral
hemorrhage; but only in one subtype of ischemic stroke: thrombotic
stroke. The researchers concluded, "The results of our case-control study
suggest that erythrocyte omega-3 PUFAs may protect against hemorrhagic stroke and ischemic stroke, particularly in the case of small-artery
occlusion [thrombotic stroke]" (Park, 2009).

DHA HELPS RECOVERY FROM STROKE

Another interesting finding about fish oil and stroke is that a 2010 study showed fish oil may help to limit or prevent brain damage following a stroke, if given within five hours after the stroke. This research has been published by Drs. N. Bazan and L. Belayev at Louisiana State University Health Sciences Center and their colleagues in a series of reports during 2010 and 2011.

DHA is the most prominent fatty acid in the brain. To determine how DHA might be effective in stroke treatment and recovery, the researchers compared DHA and saline administered intravenously at three, four, five, and six hours after the onset of an induced stroke in rats. Magnetic resonance imaging (MRI), a brain scanning technique, showed that neurological deficits were reduced by the administration of DHA. It also reduced swelling and facilitated a faster, fuller neurological recovery. The area of destroyed tissue was reduced by an average of 59 percent at five hours. Bazan remarked, "Docosahexaenoic acid of fish oil is a powerful therapeutic agent that can protect brain tissue and promote stroke recovery, even when treatment is delayed by up to five hours" (Belayev, 2011).

In a 2010 report, the research team examined the effectiveness of DHA in protecting nerve cells in acute ischemic stroke, studied the therapeutic window, and investigated whether DHA administration after an ischemic stroke is able to salvage injured brain tissue. Analysis showed that DHA treatment potentiates neuroprotectin D1 (NPD1) synthesis, a neuroprotective docosanoid with potent anti-inflammatory properties, three days after a stroke. DHA administration thus provides neurological recovery, reduces tissue damage and brain swelling, and activates protectin synthesis in the brain when administered up to five hours after experimental stroke in rats (Belayev, 2010). Protectins, which we have dealt with in a previous chapter, are substances made in the body from EPA and DHA that have protective effects on nerve cells.

Supporting evidence comes from researchers at the Université Laval in Canada in a 2011 study that showed that feeding mice a diet rich in DHA for three months significantly reduced the severity of a stroke by 25 percent (Lalancette, 2011). Their study confirmed that the consumption of DHA creates an anti-inflammatory and protective environment in the brain that mitigates damage following a stroke. In their study, mice that were genetically predisposed to stroke were divided into three groups: One group was fed a control diet, the second group was fed a diet with low levels of DHA, and the third group was fed a DHA super-enriched diet. The daily dose of DHA in the third group was about 0.7 grams of DHA per kilogram of body weight per day. The study researchers point out that given a consumption of 2,000 calories per day on average for humans, this high dose would represent approximately between 2.5 and 3 grams of DHA/EPA per day, which is still reasonable. Laboratory mice eat more than humans relative to their body weight and have a much higher metabolism rate; therefore, extrapolation of dosage from across species is difficult. Following three months of intervention, the researchers reported that the high-DHA group had lower levels of pro-inflammatory compounds, including COX-2 and interleukin (IL)-1beta in the blood. COX-2 and IL-1beta are enzymes that are used to convert fatty acids in cell membranes into eicosanoids. The data are promising, even if we cannot directly transfer the results from mice and rats to humans. We consequently can only recommend following our general recommendation of increasing your daily intake of EPA and DHA to at least 1 gram.

Clinically, fish consumption and EPA/DHA supplementation have been found to reduce the risk of having a stroke, and DHA in particular is important for recovering from a stroke. In fact, DHA is extremely important for brain function and brain health as we will discuss in the next chapters.

Fetal and Infant Neurodevelopment

esearch on omega-3, long-chain polyunsaturated fatty acids (LC-PUFAs) in brain and mental function is broadening rapidly. The necessity of a sufficient daily intake of EPA and, in particular, DHA is maybe even more important when considering brain health, than with respect to heart health!

HOW EPA AND DHA SUPPORT BRAIN DEVELOPMENT

The brain and nerve cells (neurons) have the second highest concentration of fatty acids after adipose (fat) tissue. Most of the dry weight of the brain is lipid (fat) because brain activity depends greatly upon the functions provided by lipid membranes. The brain is 60 percent fats, and DHA is the major structural fat in the brain and retina of the eye, accounting for up 97 percent of the omega-3 fats in the brain and up to 93 percent of the omega-3 fats in the retina. The retina is considered part of the brain, and vision would not be possible without the presence of DHA (more on the role of DHA in vision in Chapter 15).

DHA is the primary fatty acid in nerve cell membranes. The critical role of fatty acids in cell membranes has been discussed in Chapter 2. Less than optimal amounts of DHA in nerve cell membranes affect brain function by compromising membrane receptors, ion channels, and enzymes (properties involved in the transmission of signals between other nerve cells), as well as altering the signals carried by compounds derived from EPA and DHA that influence cognitive processes and other important brain actions. Psychiatric and neurological disorders are often associated with low brain omega-3 levels. As we will discuss in Chapter 12, emerging evidence suggests that regular consumption of EPA and DHA may be beneficial in reducing the severity of several mental conditions such as Alzheimer's disease, depression, and bipolar disorder. In children, improvements due to the consumption of EPA and DHA have been reported in attention deficit hyperactivity disorder (ADHD) and dyslexia. Caution is warranted, however, because data are as yet inconsistent and do not permit firm conclusions.

Important from the Very Beginning

EPA and DHA are essential for healthy fetal and infant brain development. The greatest dependence on dietary DHA occurs in the fetus during the last third of pregnancy and in the infant during the first three months after birth. At this time the infant's brain grows very rapidly. The brain is the most metabolically active organ in the body and at that age uses more than 50 percent of the body's energy, whereas the adult brain uses approximately 20 percent. It is during this period that brain synapses (conduits for relaying information between cells) are forming most rapidly, and an infant's demand for DHA exceeds the capacity of the body's enzymes to synthesize it from alpha-linolenic acid (ALA). The additional requirements are fulfilled by mechanisms believed to involve DHA absorption from the mother's placenta. DHA supplementation is especially important for premature infants as they have low adipose tissue reserves.

In pregnancy and early infant development, EPA and DHA are beneficial for the following:

- Important in pregnancy for transferring DHA to developing fetus

- Healthy development of the eyes and infant visual function

- Proper development of the brain and improved neurological development

- Immune system health in the infant

- Reduced risk of premature and underweight births

- Important in lactation for continual transference of DHA to baby via breast milk

During pregnancy, the developing fetus obtains omega-3 fatty acids from the mother. After birth, the infant must obtain them from breast milk or from formula supplemented with DHA. Since EPA and DHA are not present in soy, the main component of most infant formulas, some manufacturers have started supplementing their product with DHA. Breastfeeding is the best source of EPA and DHA, as well as most nutrients for the newborn—especially if the mother is well nourished and has an adequate intake of DHA. However, if formula substitutes must be used, it is wise to ensure that they contain DHA. In 2007 a panel of perinatal and newborn medical experts developed guidelines for the amount of DHA and infant formula should provide . . . brain development (see the inset below).

BREAST MILK IS BEST, BUT IF YOU CHOOSE FORMULA...

The use of omega-3 LC-PUFAs in infant formulas has been reviewed and supported by the U.S. Food and Drug Administration (FDA), the National Academy of Sciences, the Food and Agriculture Organization, the American Dietetic Association and the Dietitians of Canada, the World Health Organization, the World Association of Perinatal Medicine, and more than a dozen other global organizations.

Recommendations and guidelines for perinatal medicine have been developed by a team of nineteen experts from eleven countries who reviewed the then available research and recommendations on DHA and omega-6 arachidonic acid (AA) in 2007 and evaluated the body of research exploring how DHA and AA affect infant brain and eye development (Koletzko, 2008). The review team, which included experts from Italy, France, Germany, Spain, and the United Kingdom, concluded that both DHA and AA should be added to infant formula in order to provide formula-fed infants these important nutrients at a comparable rate to their breastfed counterparts.

The guidelines recommend that pregnant women should aim for a DHA intake of at least 200 mg a day. The DHA content of formulas should make between 0.2 and 0.5 percent of fatty acids (noting that 0.2 percent is the minimum level necessary to see functional developmental benefits). The experts also recommended an equal amount of AA.

For more information on the recommendations and guidelines, see: the World Association of Perinatal Medicine (www.wapm.info), the Early Nutrition Academy (www.metabolic-programming.org), and the Child Health Foundation (www.kindergesundheit.de).

This same panel of perinatal and newborn medical experts also compiled guidelines for pregnant or breastfeeding women. The guidelines recommend that pregnant women should aim for a DHA intake of at least 200 milligrams (mg) a day. The experts also recommended an equal amount of arachidonic acid (AA, an important and essential fatty acid in the brain). They recommended that this dietary supply of DHA and AA should continue during the second six months of life, but they did not at that time have enough information to recommend exact amounts.

In March 2010, the scientific opinion of the European Food Safety Authority Panel (EFSA) on Dietetic Products, Nutrition, and Allergies (NDA) regarding dietary reference values (DRVs) for fats, including PUFAs, was published. The opinion set an adequate intake (AI) level for DHA for infants and young children, and stated "small amounts of DHA may be needed for optimal growth and development of infants and children," including 20–50 mg per day for infants zero to six months of age (EFSA, 2010). In our opinion, this is far too low a recommendation.

Helps Develop Neurological Function

Not many studies have examined the overall effect of maternal fish intake—and thereby the intake of the omega-3 LC-PUFAs EPA and DHA—during pregnancy on child development or examined whether the developmental benefits of maternal fish intake are greater in infants breastfed for a shorter duration. An exception is the Danish National Birth Cohort study of 25,446 children born to mothers participating in a prospective population-based cohort study, including pregnant women enrolled between 1997 and 2002. Mothers reported child development by a standardized interview, which was used to generate developmental scores at ages six and eighteen months. Higher maternal fish intake and greater duration of breastfeeding were associated with higher child developmental scores at eighteen months for the highest versus the low-est quintile of fish intake, and for breastfeeding for ten months or more compared with breastfeeding for less than one month (Oken, 2008).

A study of 416 children from the Influences of Lifestyle-Related Factors on the Immune System and the Development of Allergies in Childhood (LISAplus) birth cohort from Munich found that a 1 percent increase in DHA in umbilical cord blood (measured at birth) was associated with fewer behavioral difficulties when the children were assessed at age ten (Kohlboeck, 2011). In an intervention study from Australia, the use of DHA-rich fish oil capsules compared with vegetable oil capsules during pregnancy did however not result in improved cognitive and language development in their offspring during early childhood (Makrides, 2010).

With a growing body of science on this subject, there will be con-flicting studies that will require additional studies for clarity. The use of different methodologies and unknown confounding variables can mask the true effects. However, this is a very important area of research that should be pursued.

Enhances Immunity

DHA supplementation by pregnant women may help to enhance the infants' immune systems. A study at Emory University published in the journal *Pediatrics* reported that mothers taking 400 mg of DHA had babies who overcame colds faster than babies with mothers not taking DHA supplements. At one month, the DHA group experienced 26 per-cent, 15 percent, and 30 percent shorter duration of cough, phlegm, and wheezing, respectively. At three months, infants in the DHA group spent 14 percent less time ill. At six months, infants in the DHA group experienced shorter duration of fever, nasal secretion, difficulty breathing, rash, and other illness by 20 percent, 13 percent, 54 percent, 23 percent, and 25 percent, respectively (Imhoff, 2010).

A 2012 study at the Faculty of Medicine, University of Southampton, Southampton, United Kingdom, suggests that increasing oily fish intake during pregnancy modifies neonatal immune responses. In the study, 123 women were randomly assigned to continue their habitual diet, which was low in oily fish, or to consume two portions of salmon per week (providing 3.45 grams of EPA and DHA) from twenty weeks' gestation until delivery. Umbilical cord blood samples were analyzed for omega-3 LC-PUFAs, IgE concentrations (an antibody formed as part of an allergic response), and immunologic responses. Infants were clinically evaluated at age six months. The researchers found that increasing salmon intake by a couple of servings per week during the third trimester of pregnancy improved immune system health in the infants (Noakes, 2012).

Lower Risk of Premature Birth, Obesity, and Heart Disease

Several studies have found that a high omega-3 intake during pregnancy decreases the risk of giving birth to premature babies! In one study, Norwegian researchers investigated how maternal intakes of seafood and omega-3 supplements were associated with infant birth weight, length, and head circumference. The study population included 62,099 participants in the Norwegian Mother and Child Cohort Study. The mothers answered a food-frequency questionnaire with detailed questions about intake of seafood and omega-3 supplements midway through their pregnancies. The data were matched to their baby's measurements at birth. Total seafood intake was positively associated with birth weight and head circumference (Brantsaeter, 2012).

Another study suggests that increased EPA/DHA intake and reduced omega-6 intake during pregnancy may lower the risk of future obesity in children. Researchers assessed mid-pregnancy intake of DHA and EPA and omega-6 fatty acids. They also evaluated maternal plasma fatty acid levels and umbilical cord levels of EPA, DHA, and omega-6. The children involved in the study were then assessed at age three to determine body mass index (BMI) and skin fold measurements. It was found that the odds of obesity in three-year-olds were between two and four times higher when cord blood had a high ratio of omega-6 to the omega-3 fatty acids EPA and DHA. The odds of childhood obesity were 32 percent lower when maternal intake of EPA and DHA was high (Donahue, 2011).

Omega-3s may also have a role in preventing heart disease in adults who were small at birth. Impaired fetal growth is an independent cardiovascular risk factor and is associated with arterial wall thickening in children. This study followed 616 children born at term, recruited from maternity hospitals in Sydney, Australia, who were also taking part in the Childhood Asthma Prevention Study. They were randomly assigned to receive either a 500-mg-daily fish oil supplement or canola-based margarines and cooking oil (omega-3 group), or a 500-mg-daily sunflower oil supplement and omega-6 fatty acid-rich margarines and cooking oil (control group), from the start of bottle-feeding or six months of age until five years of age. At age eight, the children were tested for the presence of arterial wall thickening, an indicator of early cardiovascular disease. In the control group, fetal growth was inversely associated with arterial wall thickening, but this was prevented in the omega-3 group! The authors concluded that the inverse association of fetal growth with arterial wall thickness in childhood can be prevented by dietary omega-3 fatty acid supplementation over the first five years of life (Skilton, 2012).

SPECIAL ISSUES AND CONCERNS

EPA and DHA dietary supplements are purified and do not contain harmful levels of methylmercury, polychlorinated biphenyls (PCBs) and other health-threatening environmental toxins in fish. In the past, there has been concern about pregnant women eating too much possibly contaminated fish—especially methylmercury, which is found in trace amounts in nearly all fish. In 2001 and again in 2004, the U.S Food and Drug Administration (FDA) advised pregnant women to limit their weekly seafood consumption. The FDA's advisory stemmed from concern that eating more fish could impair brain development by exposing the developing fetus to dangerously high levels of methylmercury.

In the two mercury health advisories, the FDA advised pregnant women and women who were thinking of becoming pregnant to eat no more than 12 ounces, or about two 6-ounce servings of fish per week. They recommended consuming no more than 6 ounces of albacore (white) tuna per week and no shark, mackerel, swordfish, or tilefish. These fish are known to contain high levels of methylmercury.

A 2007 National Institutes of Health study stated that pregnant women who limit their fish consumption to recommended government levels may be doing their unborn babies more harm than good. Researchers found that women who ate less than 12 ounces of fish or other seafood per week while pregnant were more likely to have children with verbal and other developmental delays than women who ate more than 12 ounces each week. The study comprised 11,875 pregnant women and found that maternal seafood intake of less than 340 grams (12 ounces) per week was associated with increased risk of their children being in the lowest quartile for verbal intelligence quotient (IQ) compared with children born to mothers who consumed more than 340 grams per week (Hibbeln, 2007). Because contamination levels may fluctuate and recommendations may vary over time, many people prefer fish oils and fish oil supplements that are highly purified and virtually free from methylmercury and PCBs.

COGNITIVE BENEFITS THROUGHOUT LIFE

In the coming chapters, we will discuss the considerable roles of DHA and EPA on brain function in children and adults. They have a major impact on us and our mental well-being, as well as on reducing the costs to our healthcare systems. While there are supplements available that contain either DHA alone or EPA alone, please keep in mind that both EPA and DHA are important brain nutrients. If you choose to boost your DHA intake with a supplement containing DHA alone, it is advisable to also include ample EPA in your dietary and supplement program.

11

Memory and Cognition

You probably have heard the adage that fish is brain food. Whoever started that old bromide must have been a fish eater because he or she was right. Eating enough EPA- and DHA-containing fish may make you smarter or at least slow your loss of cognitive ability with age. Studies are providing evidence to support this wisdom of the ages, which appears to hold true for growing and aging brains alike. Being primary constituents of cell membranes, EPA and DHA in healthy levels can help stimulate the formation of new nerve cells and the regeneration of existing cells. There is now fairly substantial evidence linking greater dietary intake of these omega-3, long-chain polyunsaturated fatty acids (LC-PUFAs) to better early brain development and lowered risk of cognitive disorders in late life.

HOW EPA AND DHA IMPROVE LEARNING AND COGNITIVE PERFORMANCE

One such study in 2005 at Harvard looked at 135 mothers and their infants and found that the more fish the mothers ate during their second trimesters, the better their infants did on cognition tests when they were six months old. Overall, babies' scores on the tests climbed by 4 points for each weekly serving of fish their mothers had during the second trimester. Scores were highest among infants of mothers who consumed more than two servings of fish a week (Oken, 2005).

A randomized, double-blind Norwegian study examined the effect of

133

supplementing pregnant and lactating women with omega-3 LC-PUFAs in the form of cod liver oil on mental development of the children, compared with maternal supplementation with omega-6 LC-PUFAs (corn oil). The women were recruited in week eighteen of their pregnancy to take 10 milliliters (mL) of cod liver oil or corn oil until three months after delivery. The cod liver oil contained 1,183 milligrams (mg) per 10 mL of DHA and 803 mg/10 mL of EPA. The corn oil contained 4,747 mg/10 mL of omege-6 linoleic acid (LA) and 92 mg/10 mL omega-3 alpha-linolenic acid (ALA). The amount of fat-soluble vitamins (vitamin A and vitamin D) was identical in the two oils. A total of 341 mothers took part in the study until giving birth. All infants of these women were scheduled for assessment of cognitive function at six and nine months of age. Children who were born to mothers who had taken the cod liver oil during pregnancy and lactation scored higher on the IQ testing at four years of age as compared with children whose mothers had taken the corn oil (Helland, 2003).

In 2000 a questionnaire that included dietary information was mailed to 18,158 high school students, who were fifteen years old and living in Sweden. The aim of the study was to evaluate the association between fish intake and academic grades. The study found that grades were higher in students who consumed fish once a week compared with those who ate fish less than once a week. Grades were even higher in students who consumed fish more than once a week. When stratified for parents' education, there were still higher grades among students with frequent fish intake in all educational groups. Frequent fish intake among school-age children may thus provide benefits in terms of academic achievement (Kim, 2010).

Clinical Studies with Fish Consumption

Some mental functions such as verbal ability, some numerical abilities, and general knowledge don't decline all that much over our lifetimes, but other mental capabilities can decline from middle age onward, or even earlier. The latter include aspects of memory, executive functions, processing speed, and reasoning—all of which are important for carrying out everyday activities. In normal cognitive aging, no physical underlying cause is at work, as there is in people who meet the criteria for dementia or any of the varieties of mild cognitive impairment.

A 2005 prospective cohort study called the Chicago Housing and Aging Project, or CHAP, published in the *Archives of Neurology,* looked at the cognitive effects of fish consumption in 3,718 adults. It found that elderly people who ate fish at least once a week did better on tests of memory and mental acuity than their peers who did not, and they also had a 10 percent slower decline in mental skills each year (Morris, 2005).

In April 2007, a Dutch study published in the *American Journal of Clinical Nutrition* examined the intake of omega-3 fatty acids on cognitive decline. The researchers studied the associations between the intake of EPA and DHA from fish and other foods and subsequent five-year cognitive decline in 210 men between the ages of seventy and eighty-nine. They found that fish consumers had significantly less cognitive decline over a five-year period than did non-consumers. A direct relationship was observed between EPA/DHA intake and level of cognitive decline. The researchers used a common measure of cognition called the Mini-Mental State Examination (MMSE), which has a top score of 30 points. Men who did not consume fish had a subsequent cognitive decline of 1.2 points, which was four times the decline in men who consumed fish (0.3 points). The Dutch researchers remarked, "This study showed that fish consumption in older men was associated with less subsequent five-year cognitive decline than was no fish consumption. Furthermore, a dose-response relation was noted between the combined intake of the omega-3 fatty acids EPA and DHA and cognitive decline, which suggests that a higher intake of EPA and DHA was associated with less cognitive decline." They concluded, "A moderate intake of EPA and DHA may postpone cognitive decline in elderly men. The current study provides evidence that a combined daily intake of 400 mg EPA and DHA [similar to six servings of 140 grams of lean fish per week (a total of 850 grams) or 1 serving of 140 grams of fatty fish (such as mackerel and herring) per week] is associated with less subsequent cognitive decline in elderly men" (Van Gelder, 2007).

Later that year in November, two observational studies were published in the same journal. Each study indicated that fish intake, particularly the consumption of omega-3 fatty acids in fish, could improve cognitive performance. In the first, a Norwegian study of more than 2,000 men and women, ages seventy to seventy-four, found that those who consumed more than 10 grams (0.35 ounces) of fish per day had significantly better test scores and a lower incidence of poor cognitive performance than those who consumed less than 10 grams of fish per day. The more fish consumed, the greater the effect. The best scores occurred in people who consumed about 75 grams (2.6 ounces) of fish per day (Nurk, 2007). In the second study, Dutch researchers studied 404 people between the ages of fifty and seventy, and found that higher baseline concentrations of omega-3 fatty acids were associated with a lower decline in several speed-related cognitive tests over a three-year span (Dullemeijer, 2007).

In a study published in the *American Journal of Clinical Nutrition* the following year, L. Whalley and his U.K. colleagues examined the content of omega-3 fatty acids in red blood cell membranes and cognitive changes in late midlife. They found that the total omega-3 PUFAs and specifically DHA concentrations in red blood cells were associated with enduring benefits for cognition in people between the ages of sixty-four and sixty-eight (Whalley, 2008). In this study researchers followed up on 120 people for whom IQ test scores were available from age eleven. In the first follow-up at age sixty-two, researchers drew blood samples and administered a series of cognitive tests. The tests were administered again when the participants were sixty-six and sixty-eight. Those with higher blood levels of omega-3 PUFAs consistently scored higher on the cognitive performance tests.

Clinical Studies with Fish Oil Supplements

The preceding studies were based on fish intake. As the body of science grew, it provided support for conducting clinical studies with EPA/DHA supplementation. In 2010, a randomized, double-blind, placebo-controlled, clinical study (the gold standard among studies for providing clear evidence of cause and effect) was conducted at nineteen U.S. clinical sites. The research showed that "DHA improved learning and memory function in age-related, cognitive decline and is a beneficial supplement that supports cognitive health with aging."

In this study, a total of 485 healthy people over the age of fifty-five were given a battery of standard memory tests and then randomly assigned to receive 900 mg per day of DHA or a placebo for twenty-four weeks. The researchers found that people who were taking the DHA supplement made significantly fewer errors than those taking the placebo. DHA supplementation was also associated with improved immediate and delayed verbal recognition memory scores. Over the six-month period, blood DHA levels doubled and correlated with improved scores in the DHA group (Yurko-Mauro, 2010).

Also in 2010, researchers studied the possible association between omega-3 PUFAs in blood phospholipids and cognitive functioning in mid-life adults. Participants were 280 community volunteers between the ages of thirty-five and fifty-four who had no major neuropsychiatric disorders and were not taking fish oil supplements. Their blood levels of ALA, EPA, and DHA were measured and then correlated with their results from a battery of neuropsychological tests that assess five major dimensions of cognitive functioning. Participants with the highest blood levels of DHA performed better on tests of nonverbal reasoning and mental flexibility, working memory, and vocabulary than their cohorts with lower DHA levels. Neither EPA nor ALA was notably related to any of the five tested dimensions of cognitive performance—only DHA was associated with major aspects of cognitive performance. These findings suggest that DHA is important to brain health throughout a person's life (Muldoon, 2010).

MILD COGNITIVE IMPAIRMENT

Mild cognitive impairment (MCI) describes the intermediate phase in the continuum of cognitive decline between normal aging-related changes in cognitive function and dementia, an organic disease or a disorder of the brain. PUFA levels are altered in adults with both cognitive decline and depression. Depression frequently co-exists with MCI and may increase its progression to dementia. We will discuss dementia more fully in Chapter 12 and depression in Chapter 13.

In 2011 Australian researchers investigated the associations between omega-3 and omega-6 PUFAs, and cognition, memory, and depression in fifty adults over the age of sixty-five with MCI and twenty-nine healthy controls. Memory, depressive symptoms, and PUFAs (percent of total fatty acids) were assessed. EPA levels were lower in the adults with MCI than in the healthy controls, and omega-6 PUFAs were higher in those with MCI. Higher omega-6 PUFA levels also predicted poorer mental health. Adults with MCI had higher depression scores, leading the researchers to conclude that depressive symptoms associated with elevated omega-6 PUFA may contribute to cognitive decline in this population (Milte, 2011).

In 2011 the Singapore Longitudinal Aging Study examined the association between omega-3 PUFA supplement intake and cognitive decline in an older Chinese population. The study involved 1,475 Chinese adults over age fifty-five, who did not have dementia upon enrollment. Questionnaires administered at the beginning of the study were analyzed for the frequency of omega-3 PUFA supplement use. Cognitive performance was evaluated at enrollment and one and a half years later. The researchers found that compared to those who did not take a daily omega-3 PUFA supplement, those who did supplement had a 63 percent lower risk of cognitive decline. The researchers concluded that daily omega-3 PUFA supplement consumption was independently associated with less cognitive decline in elderly Chinese (Gao, 2011).

Not many intervention studies in people with MCI have been performed, but in 2011 a six-month, randomized, controlled trial on the effects of EPA versus DHA on depressive symptoms, quality of life, memory, and executive function in older adults with MCI was published in *British Journal of Nutrition*. Depressive symptoms, as we mentioned, may increase the risk of progressing from MCI to dementia. The aim of the study was to investigate the benefits of supplementing a diet with DHA and EPA for depressive symptoms, quality of life, and cognition in elderly people with MCI. A total of fifty people aged sixty-five years or older with MCI were chosen to receive a supplement rich in EPA, DHA, or the omega-6 PUFA linoleic acid (LA). Compared with the LA group, depression scale scores improved in the EPA and DHA groups, as did verbal fluency in the DHA group. Improved depression scale scores were correlated with increased DHA plus EPA, and improved self-reported physical health was associated with increased DHA (Sinn, 2011).

SLOW YOUR LOSS OF COGNITIVE ABILITY

There are other studies, but these serve to give you an overview of the importance of EPA and DHA for brain function and cognitive ability. Remember, both EPA and DHA are important to brain health. As we pointed out in the preceding chapter, supplements of DHA alone and EPA alone are available and are fine to use, but it is advisable to include both in your dietary and supplementation program.

We will discuss mood and depression in Chapter 13, but first let's discuss the important role of EPA and DHA in reducing the risk of dementia, particularly Alzheimer's, the most common degenerative brain disease as the population ages.

CHAPTER 12

Alzheimer's Disease and Dementias

ognitive decline, as we just discussed, is closely intertwined with other brain disorders, especially with depression and dementia. In some cases, cognitive decline progresses to mild cognitive impairment, which is not only a risk factor for dementia but also a problem in itself. Yet, on the continuum of cognitive decline, where is the edge of risk between normal aging-related changes in cognitive function and dementia?

BEYOND NORMAL AGING

Dementia is any deterioration of intellectual faculties beyond normal aging such as memory, concentration, and judgment, resulting from an organic disease or a disorder of the brain, while Alzheimer's disease (AD) is a specific dementia. To be classified as dementia, there must be a decline in memory and in at least one of the following cognitive abilities severe enough to interfere with daily life:

- Ability to generate coherent speech or understand spoken or written language;

- Ability to recognize or identify objects, assuming intact sensory function;

- Ability to execute motor activities, assuming intact motor abilities, sensory function, and comprehension of the required task; and

- Ability to think abstractly, to make sound judgments, and to plan and carry out complex tasks.

When your authors were young, AD was rare. It was not known medically until German neurologist Alois Alzheimer described it in 1906. We remember when our friends were diagnosed with this then rare and horrible disease and how incredulous it seemed that they then did not even recognize us as long-time friends. Now, virtually everyone knows of several people suffering from AD. The cause of this tragic increase in this terribly debilitating disorder is not known, but it is curious that is has occurred simultaneously with the decline in dietary EPA and DHA.

The National Alzheimer's Project Act (NAPA) was signed into U.S. law in January 2011. This legislation aims to create a national strategic plan to address and overcome the rapidly escalating crisis of Alzheimer's. That same year, the Alzheimer's Association reported that there were 5.4 million people in the United States living with AD and it projected that AD will triple or quadruple by 2050. In January 2012, the Department of Health and Human Services announced the framework NAPA intended to implement to prevent and effectively treat AD by 2025.

According to a 2010 report from the Centers for Disease Control and Prevention, AD is the sixth-leading cause of death, accounting for 83,308 deaths annually in the United States after heart disease (595,444), cancer (573,855), chronic lower respiratory diseases (137,789), stroke and other cerebrovascular diseases (129,180), and accidents (118,043). The direct and indirect costs of AD and other dementias in the U.S. population now amount to more than $183 billion each year (more than heart disease and cancer put together), and, if not contained, could soar to $1 trillion a year by 2050. Medicare costs for the oldest are estimated to increase sixfold by the year 2040.

Yes, today, AD is fairly common, as is EPA/DHA deficiency. AD and EPA/DHA undernourishment are indeed strongly related, but we are not implying that one is the direct cause of the other. However, there seems to be at least an indirect relationship regarding the prevention of AD, rather than a treatment for the disease.

HOW EPA AND ESPECIALLY DHA MAY HELP PREVENT DEMENTIAS

Several studies have reported that the risk of developing a dementia such as Alzheimer's disease is inversely related to the intake of omega-3, long-chain polyunsaturated fatty acids (LC-PUFAs). Fourteen in seventeen epidemiological or cohort studies show a significant benefit of elevated omega-3 PUFA intake or blood levels in reducing the incidence of dementia found on first examination (prevalent dementia), the risk of cognitive decline, or the development of dementia during the study (incident dementia).

Early Substantive Findings

Interest in the potential neuroprotective effects of omega-3 PUFAs was first aroused by a 1997 study by Dr. S. Kalmijn and other Dutch researchers, who found an inverse relationship between the amount of fish eaten and an increased risk for AD and other dementias. Fish consumption was inversely related to dementia with a 60 percent reduced risk, and in particular to a 70 percent reduced risk of AD (Kalmijn, 1997). Their study also suggested that a high-saturated fat and cholesterol intake increases the risk of dementia, whereas fish consumption may decrease this risk. However, in 2002, after analysis of follow-up data obtained from these participants, the researchers found that the association did not hold. It is felt that the study initially failed to establish rigorous parameters.

That there is a relationship between dietary omega-3 LC-PUFAs from fish was most convincingly shown in a cohort of the Framingham Heart Study, which found that a mean DHA intake of 180 milligrams (mg) per day was associated with a significant reduction in the risk of developing all-cause dementia. The study examined blood levels of DHA in 899 participants at the beginning of the study and followed them for approximately nine years. During that time, 99 cases of dementia were observed. Those participants having higher blood levels of DHA at the start of the study had a reduced incidence of dementia. Men and women whose blood DHA levels were in the top quartile of all participants were 47 percent less likely to develop any dementia and 39 percent less likely to develop AD (Schaefer, 2006). This study was the first prospective analysis to assess the predictive value of blood DHA content in the occurrence of dementia and AD. Its strengths lie in its prospective design, its long follow-up period (nine years on average), the size of the sample, and the analysis of dietary data along with the direct assessment of the association between dementia and plasma phospholipid fatty acid content.

A number of large population-based studies from the Netherlands, Norway, France, and Italy have since found the same relationship between increased fish- and omega-3 LC-PUFA consumption and decreased AD risk, which consequently seems solidly documented.

Prevent Formation of Plaques

A leading theory of the cause of AD is that plaques are formed from beta-amyloid, a protein that is toxic to nerve cells. Beta-amyloid plaques are clumps of misfolded protein fragments. Abnormal accumulation of beta-amyloid is an early occurrence in AD development. When levels of beta-amyloid become excessive, large areas of brain cells are destroyed and brain function is impaired. This abnormal accumulation of beta-amyloid is associated with defects and tangles in the tau proteins of brain neurons. Tau proteins are important for stabilizing nerve cells and defective tau proteins are associated with dementias including AD. The plaques can affect nerve cells in almost any area of the brain and result in deficits in thought control, memory, language, and other mental abilities.

EPA and DHA are thought to alter toxic beta-amyloid formation by producing neuroprotectins (substances that protect brain cells) that lead to the formation of harmless amyloid peptides. Although these neuroprotectins have not been shown to undo amyloid plaques that are already formed, they have essential functional roles and pathophysiological functions in the brain, which may be protective (Bazan, 2005).

An important literature review in 2010 by Drs. G. A. Jicha and the late W. R. Markesbery of the Sanders Brown Center on Aging at the University of Kentucky College of Medicine, Lexington, explains several probable mechanisms that enable EPA and DHA to influence the accumulation and formation of amyloid plaque. The amyloid theory of AD is based on the early formation of toxic beta-amyloid fragments from larger amyloid precursor proteins (APP). Studies suggest that EPA and DHA reduce the formation of these plaques by: 1) facilitating the interaction of enzymes (called alpha-secretases) that cleave APP to produce (smaller) non-toxic fragments; 2) shielding the cleavage site where enzymes (called gamma-secretases) function; 3) serving as a trap for free radicals that damage the protein complex important for the regulation of normal gamma-secretase function; and 4) directly inhibiting beta-amyloid formation (Jicha, 2010). Support for EPA/DHA's role in reducing beta-amyloid was confirmed in a study, which found that a high intake of dietary omega-3 combined with one additional gram of omega-3 per day lowered blood levels of beta-amyloid by 20–30 percent (Gu, 2012). Also, DHA significantly increases a protein in neurons called *LR11*. Low levels of LR11 are known to increase the production of beta-amyloid plaques and may be a significant genetic cause of AD (Ma, 2007).

May Inhibit Inflammatory Processes in Brain Cells

There is also evidence to suggest that inflammation is somehow involved in the pathogenesis of AD. The exact role(s) of inflammation in the pathogenesis of dementia including AD is still not fully understood. Although some studies have been able to demonstrate the presence of activated microglia (a marker of the brain's immune response) in individuals with probable AD, a number of prospective clinical trials evaluating the use of available drugs that target various aspects of the immune system have only produced marginal benefit. However, the anti-inflammatory roles of EPA and DHA take different routes and could possibly lead to better results.

One compound of special interest is neuroprotectin D1 (NPD1). NPD1 is generated from DHA and has potent inflammatory-resolving and neuroprotective activity. NPD1 reduces the release of toxic peptides from aging human brain cells and is severely depleted in the AD brain. Recent studies in mice show that NPD1 significantly reduces both the chemical messengers that initiate inflammation and amyloid peptide formation, underscoring the potential of DHA to rescue human brain cells in early stages of degeneration (Zhao, 2011).

Preserve Brain Volume

At the 97th annual meeting of the Radiological Society of North America, held in December 2011, Dr. C. Raji and his colleagues at the University of Pittsburg School of Medicine reported that people who consumed baked or broiled fish at least one time per week had better preservation of gray matter volume on magnetic resonance imaging (MRI) brain scan in areas at risk for AD. The study established a direct relationship between fish consumption, brain structure, and AD risk. Gray matter, also known as the cerebral cortex, is the outer layer of the brain. It is made up of specialized nerve cells involved in executive functions such as memory, attention, perceptual awareness, thought, language, and consciousness.

For the study, 260 cognitively healthy individuals were selected from the Cardiovascular Health Study. Information on fish consumption was gathered using a food-frequency questionnaire. There were 163 patients who consumed fish on a weekly basis, and the majority ate fish one to four times per week. Each patient underwent 3-D volumetric MRI scan of the brain. A brain-mapping technique that measures gray matter volume was used to model the relationship between weekly fish consumption at baseline and brain structure ten years later. The data were then analyzed to determine if gray matter volume preservation associated with fish consumption reduced risk for AD.

The study findings showed that consumption of baked or broiled fish on a weekly basis was positively associated with gray matter volume in several areas of the brain. Greater gray matter volume in relation to fish consumption reduced the risk for five-year decline to MCI or AD by almost fivefold. Raji remarked, "Consuming baked or broiled fish promotes stronger neurons in the brain's gray matter by making them larger and healthier. This simple lifestyle choice increases the brain's resistance to AD and lowers risk for the disorder." The results also demonstrated increased levels of cognition in people who ate baked or broiled fish. Dr. Raji reported, "Working memory, which allows people to focus on tasks and commit information to short-term memory, is one of the most important cognitive domains. Working memory is destroyed by Alzheimer's disease. We found higher levels of working memory in people who ate baked or broiled fish on a weekly basis, even when accounting for other factors, such as education, age, gender and physical activity" (Raji, 2011). Eating fried fish, on the other hand, was not shown to increase brain volume or protect against cognitive decline—not surprising given the similar findings in heart disease and stroke. (To learn more about the importance of fish preparation methods, see the inset on page 119.)

In the 2010 literature review mentioned earlier by Jicha and Markesbery, they concluded that "data from the cross-sectional, epidemiologic, and prospective cohort studies of the associations between dietary omega-3 PUFA intake and cognitive status have been largely positive. Dietary habits in these cohorts are likely longstanding rather than short-lived, as in a clinical trial paradigm." They also noted that "the prospective clinical trial data on omega-3 PUFA supplementation to date suggest a potentially positive effect of DHA supplementation on select persons within the study cohorts only."

FACTORS THAT INHIBIT PROTECTIVE ACTIONS OF EPA AND DHA

The relationship between EPA/DHA status and dementia is complicated by a few factors that sometimes produce studies with conflicting results. The beneficial effects of omega-3 PUFA supplementation appear to depend on the stage of the dementia, the status of a blood protein called *apolipoprotein E,* or APO-E, and confounding dietary factors like saturated and trans fats.

Stage of Dementia

In 2006, a large-scale, randomized, double-blind, placebo-controlled trial of omega-3 LC-PUFA supplementation was reported by Y. Freund-Levi and colleagues. The group studied 204 patients with mild to moderate AD. The patients received a cholinesterase inhibitor drug, a commonly prescribed AD drug, throughout the study and were also randomly assigned either 1.7 grams of DHA and 0.6 grams of EPA per day, or a placebo for six months. No significant differences in delaying the rate of cognitive decline were observed between the treated and placebo groups. However, analysis of a subgroup of mildly affected individuals showed significantly less cognitive decline compared to the placebo subgroup. Only 31 percent of the study cohort were APO-E4 non-carriers and the treatment effect of APO-E4 status was not evaluated (more about APO-E4 below). The researchers concluded, "The beneficial effects of omega-3 PUFA supplementation may be dependent on cognitive status at time of treatment intervention with those in the earliest stages of disease benefiting most" (Freund-Levi, 2006).

In 2009 another trial of EPA/DHA supplementation was reported by Y. Freund-Levi and colleagues. Thirty-five men and women between the ages of sixty-two and seventy-eight with AD were randomly assigned to a daily intake of 1.7 grams of DHA and 0.6 grams of EPA (2.3 grams total daily) or a placebo for six months. The inflammatory markers interleukin (IL)-6, tumor necrosis factor-alpha, and soluble interleukin-1 receptor type II (sIL-1RII) were analyzed in cerebral spinal fluid (CSF) and plasma at baseline and at six months. The AD markers tau protein and beta-amyloid were assessed in CSF. The researchers found no significant treatment effect of EPA or DHA on inflammatory and AD biomarkers in CSF or on inflammatory markers in plasma, nor was there any relation with APO-E. They concluded, "Treatment of AD patients with omega-3 FAs [fatty acids] for six months did not influence inflammatory or biomarkers in CSF or plasma" (Freund-Levi, 2009).

In a 2010 study, 402 individuals were randomly assigned to receive 2 grams of DHA a day or a placebo for eighteen months. In the 295 participants who completed the trial, supplementation with DHA did not slow the rate of cognitive and functional decline in patients with mild to moderate AD (Quinn, 2010). In contrast, in 2011, a prospective study with 3,294 adults from the Supplementation with Antioxidant Vitamins and Minerals Study found that cognitive complaints (often an early indicator of cognitive decline) were less frequent among the elderly who had a high EPA/DHA intake, when compared with an assessment conducted thirteen years earlier (Kesse-Guyot, 2011).

APO-E4 Gene

Some researchers have observed that the dementia protection from DHA appears to be less in individuals who carry a gene variant of the blood protein APO-E called *APO-E4*. APO-E4 is thought to increase deposits of amyloid plaque in the brain. It has also been implicated in atherosclerosis, impaired cognitive function, and reduced nerve cell repair.

APO-E4 is the largest known genetic risk factor for early-onset AD (an uncommon form of the disease that strikes people younger than sixty-five) in a variety of ethnic groups. Caucasians and Japanese who carry two copies of the APO-E4 gene variant have between ten and thirty times the risk of developing Alzheimer's by seventy-five years of age, as compared to those who are not carrying the APO-E4 gene. (It's important to note that people without APO-E4 can develop AD; however, it's just not as likely.) Many of the protective benefits of EPA and DHA from dietary and supplement interventions appear to benefit APO-E4 non-carriers but not APO-E4 carriers.

An example of the relationship among DHA, APO-E4, and AD is seen in a French study by Dr. P. Barberger-Gateau and colleagues. The investigators examined the diets of 8,085 French people from Bordeaux, Dijon, and Montpellier. They found that weekly fish consumption was associated with a reduced risk of AD and all-cause dementia only in those who were not APO-E4 carriers. The researchers also determined that a high consumption of omega-6 to omega-3 fatty acids was associated with an increased risk of all types of dementia, but again only among those who were not APO-E4 carriers (Barberger-Gateau, 2007).

In 2003 Dr. M. Morris and colleagues studied the diets of 815 subjects in the Chicago Housing and Aging Project. Their findings showed that those who consumed fish once a week or more had a 60 percent reduced risk of AD compared to those who rarely or never ate fish. Total PUFA and DHA, but not EPA intake, were associated with this reduced risk for Alzheimer's (Morris, 2003). Consumption of alpha-linolenic acid (ALA) was also protective, but only in APO-E4 carriers, in contrast to the positive effects of PUFAs seen only in APO-E4 non-carriers in the 2000 Canadian Study of Health and Aging (CHSA) study.

In 2005 the CHSA trial also examined the association of fish intake (lean versus fatty) with dementia, AD, and vascular dementia in relation to APO-E4 status in 2,233 people. The researchers reported that while consumption of lean fried fish had no protective effect, the consumption of fatty fish more than twice a week was associated with a reduced risk of dementia and AD. This effect was selective for non-carriers of the APO-E4 gene only (Huang, 2005).

In 2008, L. Whalley and colleagues reported on their study, which measured the omega-3 LC-PUFA content of red blood cell membranes and cognitive performance in 113 cognitively healthy Scottish volunteers. Fish oil supplements were equally distributed between APO-E4 carriers and non-carriers. Over the next four years a series of follow-ups were conducted. While cognitive benefits were associated with higher cell membrane levels of omega-3 LC-PUFA content, this association was only significant in APO-E4 non-carriers (Whalley, 2008).

Confounding Dietary Factors

In 2003 researchers from Dublin, Ireland, published a case-control study involving 148 patients with AD and 45 cognitively healthy controls. The researchers measured the participants' blood levels of EPA, DHA, and saturated fatty acids. While all three measurements were significantly reduced in the blood from AD patients as compared to the blood from the dementia-free group, only DHA and saturated fatty acids were associated with lower scores on the Mini-Mental State Examination (MMSE) and Clinical Dementia Rating scale (CDR), two widely used tests to screen for Alzheimer's (Tully, 2003).

Man-made trans fats seem to cause brain damage as measured by brain aging and shrinkage. A study published in 2012, led by G. L. Bowman at Oregon Health and Science University and the Linus Pauling Institute at Oregon State University, found that "junk food diets" containing high levels of trans fats may lead to brain shrinkage associated with AD (Bowman 2011). Using thirty blood biomarkers of diet, the researchers found three distinctive patterns associated with more favorable cognitive and MRI measures: 1) high levels of EPA and DHA; 2) high levels of vitamins B (B_1, B_2, B_6, folate, and B_{12}), C, D, and E; and 3) low levels of trans fats.

The third pattern characterized by high trans fat was associated with less favorable cognitive function and less total cerebral brain volume. This study involved 104 healthy elderly (with an average age of eighty-seven). MRI brain scans were performed on forty-two of the participants, with the findings that those who had high blood levels of EPA and DHA, and high blood levels of vitamins, had larger brains and those with high levels of trans fats were prone to the type of brain shrinkage associated with AD.

In addition to the studies we have cited, the few others that do not support the findings that fish oil is protective against dementias have weaknesses, such as not considering APO-E4 status and dietary intake of omega-6 PUFAs, or saturated or trans fats that are known to interfere with the availability of omega-3 PUFAs. Seventy percent of the studies (seven in ten) that considered APO-E4 status and 71 percent of the studies (five in seven) that considered dietary intake of omega-6 fatty acids and saturated and trans fats found a significant impact of these factors on the association of omega-3 PUFA status with cognitive decline or dementia.

PROTECT YOUR BRAIN

As Mom always said, fish is brain food. The overwhelming body of science shows a positive effect of EPA/DHA intake on protecting against AD and all types of dementia. Clinical trials in the future of people with moderate to severe dementia must consider not only EPA/DHA blood levels, but APO-E4, omega-6 fatty acids, and saturated and trans fat levels as well—factors that scientists now know can inhibit actions of EPA and DHA to degrade beta-amyloid buildup.

Meanwhile, we suggest that everyone consider the multitude of positive studies showing the preventive role of the omega-3 LC-PUFAs EPA and DHA in protecting against cognitive decline, including Alzheimer's disease and other dementias, and that those, in particular with mild Alzheimer's, might benefit from EPA/DHA supplementation. At a minimum, your diet should contain at least 400 mgs of EPA/DHA combined, and preferably, 1,000 mg of EPA/DHA combined, to reduce the risk of AD and dementias.

Mood and Depression

nhance your mood and feel better! Everyone likes to be in a good mood and free of depression. "Believe it or not!" as Mr. Ripley would say, your diet—especially its omega-3 long-chain polyunsaturated fatty acid (LC-PUFA) content—can affect your mood. In this chapter, we will discuss the role of these omega-3 fatty acids in everyday mood and in mood disorders.

Depression is the most common of the serious psychiatric disorders. Lifetime prevalence varies widely, from 3 percent in Japan to 17 percent in the United States. In most countries studied, the number of people who experience depression during their lives falls within an 8–12 percent range. In North America the probability of having a major depressive episode within a yearlong period is 3–5 percent for men and 8–10 percent for women. Studies have consistently shown depression to be about twice as common in women as in men, although it is not known why (Kuehner, 2003). People are most likely to suffer their first depressive episode between the ages of thirty and forty, and there is a second, smaller peak of incidence between ages fifty and sixty.

Depression is more than sadness. Depression is an illness that can become disabling or worse! It is a major cause of morbidity worldwide. Depression ranges from mild (subclinical) depression to major (clinical) depression. It is a biopsychosocial illness that includes a biochemical disorder of the brain. The causes of depression include biological, psychological, and social factors. Depression can make life difficult and profoundly agonizing. There is no good reason to allow mild depression to progress to the point of incapacitation or major depression. The good news is that fish oil can improve mood and help counter depression in its earlier stages. Even in more severe depression, fish oil supplements alone or in combination with medication, have helped many seemingly incurable patients lead normal lives.

HOW EPA AND DHA MAY COUNTER MOOD DISORDERS

EPA and DHA have been shown in several studies to have a positive effect on mental health and mood. In one study, EPA was found to be as effective as Prozac in reducing symptoms of depression (Jazayeri, 2008).

There are several mechanisms that could explain how EPA and DHA affect brain functions like mood and behavior. The fatty acid composition of a cell membrane determines its biophysical properties and influences

nerve transmission and cellular communication. Greater concentration of omega-3 LC-PUFAs in nerve cell membranes leads to greater membrane fluidity, which in turn increases the transport of the neurotransmitter serotonin, a brain chemical that is needed for brain function and is vital to nerve cells for regulating mood. These biochemical mechanisms connect EPA and DHA to a popular theory on the cause of depression called the *receptor- and neurotransmitter-based hypothesis* of depression. This hypothesis proposes that depression is the result of serotonin deficiency.

However, other biochemical mechanisms could also explain the relationship. Besides being selectively concentrated in the synaptic parts of neuronal cell membranes (areas where neve cells connect to other nerve cells), EPA and DHA are involved in the regulation of vascular and immune functions that affect the central nervous system. For example, EPA/DHA deficiencies increase the risk of debilitating diseases such as atherosclerosis and inflammatory compounds. Both inflammation and atherosclerosis have been associated with depression and could link fatty acids and depression (Maes, 1996, 1999; Alexopoulos, 1997).

The two major classifications of mood disorders are unipolar and bipolar. Unipolar disorders include mild (subclinical) depression, also known as dysthmia, and major (clinical) depression (a more serious form of depression), also known as major depressive disorder. Bipolar disorders (or manic-depressive illness, alternating episodes of depression and mania) include bipolar disorders type I and II and cyclothymic disorder (a milder form of bipolar disorder and will be discussed in Chapter 14).

Depression symptoms and classifications are often overlapping so studies tend to examine several aspects of depression at the same time. This presents a challenge for us to tease out the portions of such studies to report to you under single topics, but we'll do our best to minimize the confusion. First, let's take a quick look at the role of EPA and DHA on general everyday mood, behavior, and depression.

MOOD, BEHAVIOR, AND DEPRESSION

Interest in EPA and DHA on mood stems from their importance in brain cell membrane structure and function. In a 2002 study of fish consumption and mental health status, Drs. K. M. Silvers and K. M. Scott of the New Zealand Institute for Crop and Food Research found that fish eaters had on average a mental component score that was 8.2 points higher than non-fish eaters (Silvers, 2002). The researchers stated, "This cross-sectional survey demonstrates a significant relationship between fish intake and higher self-reported mental health status, therefore offering indirect support for the hypothesis that omega-3 polyunsaturated fatty acids may act as mood stabilisers."

In a 2007 epidemiological study of 2,416 New Zealanders fifteen years of age or older, researchers found a consistent association between high blood levels of EPA and better self-reported physical and mental well-being, and low blood levels and poorer mental and physical well-being. The researchers reported, "The results suggest a strong and consistent association between eicosapentaenoic acid [EPA] in serum phospholipids and self-reported physical well-being; the association with mental well-being is less compelling" (Crowe, 2007).

A 2008 meta-analysis by Dr. K. Appleton and colleagues evaluated the published studies on mood. The researchers reviewed the relevant evidence from a combination of eighteen epidemiological, clinical, and intervention trials. They found that most of the evidence supports a positive role for omega-3 PUFAs in countering depression, depressive symptoms, suicidal behavior, anxiety and anxiety-related disorders, and some symptoms of these disorders such as aggression, anger, and antisocial behavior. In this 2008 study, the researchers evaluated the body of science as "Epidemiological studies provide some evidence that omega-3 PUFA intake is associated with depressed mood, but not all studies have found associations. Clinical studies also provide some evidence that depression may be associated with reduced omega-3 PUFA status, although the results are inconclusive" (Appleton, 2008).

Two years later the same research group expanded their review to include seventeen additional studies, for a total of thirty-five studies, and found that "Trial evidence of the effects of omega-3 PUFAs on depressed mood has increased but remains difficult to summarize because of considerable heterogeneity [differences in design of studies]. The evidence available provides some support of a benefit of omega-3 PUFAs in individuals with diagnosed depressive illness but no evidence of any benefit in individuals without a diagnosis of depressive illness" (Appleton, 2010).

Lower Anxiety and Anger

Just how strong is the association between behavior and omega-3 LC-PUFAs? Consider the following three studies. The first study involves substance abusers.

The 2008 study of substance abusers by the New York Harbor Healthcare System found, "Adequate ω-3 [omega-3] PUFA intake via supplementation benefits substance abusers by reducing their anger and anxiety levels. The strong correlations between an increase in plasma EPA and lower anxiety scores and between an increase in plasma DHA and lower anger scores suggest a need for the further exploration of the differential responses to these two ω-3 PUFAs in different psychiatric conditions." In this small, double-blind randomized trial, twenty-two substance abusers received either 3 grams of omega-3 LC-PUFAs, or a placebo daily for three months. Blood samples and anger and anxiety tests were taken at the start and the end of the study. The researchers found that while the substance abusers' dietary intakes of omega-3 PUFAs fell below recommended dietary levels, those receiving the omega-3 LC-PUFA treatment showed significant decreases in anger and anxiety scores compared to those taking the placebo. These changes were associated with increases in blood levels of both EPA and DHA; an increase in EPA was more strongly correlated with lower anxiety scores, while an increase in DHA was more robustly correlated with lower anger scores (Buydens-Branchey, 2008).

If EPA and DHA can reduce elevated levels of anger in drug abusers, can they reduce elevated levels of anger in hardened offenders like young prisoners? Apparently so, according to at least two studies: one British and one Dutch.

In the first of the two studies, British prisoners were given either a placebo or a supplement containing vitamins, minerals, and essential fatty acids. Compared with prisoners taking the placebos, those receiving the active capsules committed an average of 26.3 percent fewer offenses. Compared to baseline measures, the effect on the 172 prisoners taking active supplements for a minimum of two weeks was an average 35.1 percent reduction of offenses, whereas those prisoners receiving the placebos showed no improvement as their offenses remained within the range of standard error (Gesch, 2002).

In the second of the two studies, researchers from the Ministry of Justice at the Hague studied the effects of food supplements on aggression, rule-breaking, and psychopathology among young Dutch prisoners. Two hundred and twenty-one prisoners, ranging in age from eighteen to twenty-five, received nutritional supplements containing vitamins, minerals, and essential fatty acids or placebos, over a period of one to three months. As in the former British study, the Dutch study reported that antisocial incidents were significantly reduced (by 34 percent) in the 115 prisoners taking the supplements, as compared to the group of 106 taking the placebo. Since the incidents reported concerned aggressive and rule-breaking behavior as observed by the prison staff, the results are considered to be promising (Zaalberg, 2010).

These results support the findings in a Japanese study of forty-one students who took either capsules containing 1.5–1.8 grams of DHA per day (seventeen girls and five boys) or control oil capsules containing 97 percent soybean oil plus 3 percent fish oil (twelve girls and seven boys) for three months. The study started at the end of summer vacation and ended in the middle of mentally stressful final exams. In the control group extra-aggression (aggression against others) was significantly increased at the end of the study as compared with that measured at the start, whereas it was not significantly changed in the DHA group (Hamazaki, 1996).

Improve Mood and Alertness

The aim of a study performed at the University of Siena in Italy was to examine the effects of omega-3 PUFAs on some cognitive and physiological parameters in healthy people. Participants were tested at the beginning of the experiment and after thirty-five days. In this period one group was supplemented with omega-3 PUFAs. Another group was supplemented with olive oil as a placebo. In each group, tests involving different types of attention (Alert, Go/No-Go, Choice and Sustained Attention) were used in each group. For each test, reaction time and several other parameters were recorded by electroencephalogram (EEG), and a mood profile (Profile of Mood States test, or POMS) was performed. The mood profile was improved in participants taking the omega-3 supplement with increased vigor and reduced anger, anxiety, and depression states. The improved mood resulted in improved reactivity as measured by a reduction in reaction time and accuracy. The authors concluded that omega-3 supplementation is associated with an improvement of attentional and physiological functions, particularly those involving complex mental processing. They found this to be a surprisingly positive outcome in healthy people (Fontani, 2005)!

Another study from Italy has parallel findings in athletes. The purpose of this study was to determine the effect of omega-3 PUFAs and policosanol supplementation on the cognitive processes involved in the control of reactivity in *karateka* (karate practitioners) engaged in attention tests. Policosanol is a mixture of a few fatty alcohols (mostly octacosanol) extracted from plants. Eighteen karateka were randomly assigned to two groups. One group (ten subjects) took the supplement of omega-3 PUFAs (2.25 grams) plus policosanol (10 milligrams) for twenty-one days, and the other group was supplemented with placebo (oleic sunflower oil) for the same period (Fontani, 2009).

The participants were tested at the beginning of the experiment, and after twenty-one and forty-two days. The experimental procedure consisted of attention test and reaction time tests. The karateka had to react by pressing a key of a computer keyboard in one of the tests and a sequence of three keys in another test in response to stimuli. For each test, the reaction time was measured and a POMS test was also administered. The researchers concluded that "Supplementation with omega-3 fatty acids plus policosanol may be effective in improving mood state and reactivity. The reaction-time reduction appears to be due to a central nervous system effect. These results are in line with previous experiments."

So it seems that a high dietary intake of omega-3 PUFAs and supplementation plays an important role in stabilizing mood and behavior, as well as increasing mental well-being. Now, let's look at major depression. Research psychiatrists, including Drs. M. Weissman and G. Klerman, have shown a dramatic jump in major depression rates with each subsequent decade of the twentieth century, and even more alarming is that the age of onset of major depression has decreased concomitantly (Klerman, 1989).

MAJOR DEPRESSION

Major depression is common, affecting about 121 million people worldwide. Everyone will at some time in their life be affected by depression—whether their own or someone else's, according to statistics. Major depression affects about 8 percent of the U.S. population ages eighteen and older in a given year. It appears to occur at similar rates in large metropolitan areas, small metropolitan areas, and non-metropolitan areas—but does vary by annual family income (the lower the income, the higher the rate of depression). One in four women will experience depression at some point in life. According to a Rand Corporation Report, depression results in more absenteeism than almost any other physical disorder and costs employers more than $51 billion per year in absenteeism and lost productivity, not including high medical and pharmaceutical bills (Miranda, 2008).

In his book *The Omega-3 Connection* (2001), psychiatrist A. L. Stoll, who is best known for his research into omega-3 fatty acids and for their role in treating depression, presents four types of evidence that validate the antidepressant effects of the omega-3s. He writes, "First, there are compelling population (epidemiological) studies linking the eating of large amounts of fish to low rates of major depression. The second line of evidence includes neurochemical studies in animals (looking at brain chemistry). The third line of evidence involves biochemical analyses of omega-3 fatty acids and related compounds in the blood of patients with major depression. Clinical evidence comprises the fourth line."

Let's look at each line of evidence and the findings that emerged.

Fish Intake and Depression

The first news of omega-3 fatty acids and depression to attract widespread attention was a 1998 report in *The Lancet* by Dr. J. Hibbeln of the National Institutes of Health. At this time it had long been observed that people who are depressed are at greater risk for heart disease. When data began showing the relationship between fish oil and decreased incidence of heart disease, Hibbeln began looking for a parallel association between fish consumption and depression. Using data from the Weismann and Klerman study and other research findings, Hibbeln confirmed an inverse relationship between fish consumption and depression incidence: the less fish a population consumed, the higher the rates of depression (Hibbeln, 1998).

Brain Chemistry and Depression

While Hibbeln was investigating the similarity between heart disease and depression and the inverse relationship with omega-3 LC-PUFAs, other researchers, including Dr. R. S. Smith at the University of Virginia, Charlottesville, were noting links between depression and the immune and inflammatory systems.

The possibility that an imbalance of omega-6 to omega-3 fatty acids and inflammation was a factor in depression was first introduced in 1991 by Smith with his macrophage theory of depression. Smith proposed that macrophages (a type of white blood cell) could secrete excessive quantities of cytokines (chemical messengers) and other inflammatory molecules (Smith, 1991). He noted that omega-3 and omega-6 fatty acids regulate these compounds. It has been established that excessive amounts of certain omega-6-derived interleukins (not balanced by appropriate amounts of omega-3 derived interleukins) can cause bouts of major depression (Smith, 1991). The regions of the brain affecting mood are greatly influenced by the powerful inflammatory cytokines interleukin-1

(IL-1), interleukin-6 (IL-6), and tumor necrosis factor. These cytokines can decrease the production of the neurotransmitter serotonin. Supplies of serotonin are also greatly affected by EPA and DHA.

Blood Levels and Depression

In 1998, researchers in the United Kingdom led by Dr. M. Peet reported that there was significant depletion of omega-3 fatty acids in the red blood cell membranes of depressed people that was not due to reduced caloric intake. They found that the severity of depression correlated negatively with membrane levels and with dietary intake of omega-3 PUFAs, especially with DHA. The researchers concluded, "Lower [levels of] omega-3 PUFAs are associated with the severity of depression" (Edwards, 1998). A number of studies confirmed these results.

The link between blood levels of fatty acids and depression was confirmed in a later epidemiological study called the Rotterdam Study. This study, led by Dr. H. Tiemeier, examined whether elderly people with depression, living in a suburb of Rotterdam, have a fatty acid composition that is different from that of nondepressed people living in the same locale. As part of the study, 3,884 adults, sixty or older, were screened for depressive symptoms. The researchers compared percentages of omega-3 and omega-6 PUFAs and their ratios between 264 adults with depressive symptoms, including 106 participants with depressive disorders, and 461 randomly selected people. They also examined whether atherosclerosis or the inflammatory response (as measured by CRP, a marker of inflammation in the body) underlies the relation between fatty acid composition and depression.

The researchers found that adults with depressive disorders had a higher ratio of total (combined) omega-6 to total omega-3 PUFAs. However, depressed subjects had a substantially altered fatty acid composition. The percentages of omega-3 PUFAs and the ratios of omega-6 to omega-3 PUFAs were significantly lower and higher, respectively, in those with depressive disorders than in control subjects (5.2 percent omega-3 PUFAs in depressed persons compared with 5.9 percent omega-3 PUFAs in non-depressed persons, and 7.2 percent omega-6/ omega-3 PUFAs in depressed persons compared with 6.6 percent omega-6/omega-3 PUFAs in non-depressed persons, respectively). This relation was not due to atherosclerosis. These findings support the concept that lower EPA and DHA are associated with increased risk of depression.

The researchers concluded, "In community-dwelling persons, fatty acid composition is related to depression. Because this relation was not secondary to inflammation, atherosclerosis, or possible co-founders, it suggests a direct effect of fatty acid composition on mood." (Tiemeier, 2003).

Clinical Studies and Depression

The first psychiatrist to publish a clinical study on the use of omega-3 fatty acids to treat various depressions appears to have been Dr. D. O. Rudin of the Eastern Pennsylvania Psychiatric Institute. Rudin used flaxseed oil, which is rich in the medium-chain omega-3 alpha-linolenic acid (ALA), in a small open-label study (where both patient and physician are aware of the substance being given) with twelve patients with a variety of depressive symptoms. Although the results of Rudin's small study are difficult to interpret, the point is that he may have been one of the first psychiatrists to investigate the link between omega-3 deficiency and depression (Rudin, 1996).

Several years earlier, Dr. Stoll, the psychopharmacologist (psychiatrist specializing in medication treatments) who we already mentioned, was becoming increasingly dismayed at the number and severity of the side effects from the drugs used to treat major depression, especially bipolar depression. Often these drugs have to be used at high dosages and/or in combination. Stoll and his colleague Dr. E. Severus started their hunt for better treatments in 1993. They did extensive computer searches of the literature (not as simple in 1993 as now) and were astonished to find the consistent benefit-to-risk ratio (best results versus least side effects) was fish oil (Stoll, 1999).

Given the safety of fish oil, they began adding it to their treatment protocols. In *The Omega-3 Connection* Stoll recounts, "I began prescribing [omega-3 fatty acids] in open-label fashion . . . for sixteen patients with treatment-resistant major depression. . . . I added a daily dosage of omega-3 fatty acids (either fish oil or flaxseed oil) to their ongoing antidepressant medication. We found the results encouraging. Five of the sixteen responded at least partially, and four of those experienced marked improvement when omega-3 was added to their ongoing antidepressant treatment. While five of sixteen (22 percent) may not seem impressive, it is important to realize these were treatment-resistant cases, where response rates are usually quite low, often well below 10 percent" (Stoll, 2001).

Encouraged by these results, Stoll and his colleagues did a formal clinical study of fish oil and both unipolar and bipolar depression. We will discuss bipolar depression in the next chapter, but this study is import-ant to our discussion of unipolar depression as well. They studied thirty manic-depressive patients and found that 64 percent of those who took 10 grams of fish oil per day for four months reported a marked improve-ment in their symptoms. By contrast, only 19 percent of those receiving the placebo improved (Stoll, 1999).

In 2006 Drs. Stoll, M. Freeman, J. Hibbeln, and eight of their col-leagues, serving on the Omega-3 Fatty Acids Sub-Committee assembled by the Committee on Research on Psychiatric Treatments of the Ameri-can Psychiatric Association, published their findings on the evidence for omega-3 PUFA treatment in *Psychiatry*. They wrote, "The preponderance of epidemiologic and tissue compositional studies supports a protective effect of omega-3 EFA intake, particularly EPA and DHA, in mood dis-orders. Meta-analysis of randomized controlled trials demonstrate a sta-tistically significant benefit in unipolar and bipolar depression" (Freeman, 2006).

A 2009 double-blind, placebo-controlled, randomized clinical trial of omega-3 supplementation in the treatment of psychological distress and depressive symptoms in middle-aged women found positive results. After eight weeks, women with psychological distress without major depressive episodes at the time of enrollment, showed changes in psychological distress and depressive scales and improved significantly more with EPA than with a placebo (Lucas, 2009).

In 2010 an Italian study of depressed older women confined to a nurs-ing home found that taking fish oil supplements for eight weeks (2,500 mg once daily, consisting of 1,670 mg of EPA and 830 mg of DHA) resulted in a remission of depression in 40.9 percent compared to 16.7 percent of those taking placebo. The study also found a statistically significant improvement in the self-assessed quality of life. The researchers concluded, "Supplementation with omega-3 LC-PUFA is efficacious in the amelioration of depressive symptoms and quality of life in the treatment of depressed elderly female patients" (Rondanelli, 2010).

In 2011 a study at the Department of Psychiatry, Leiden University Medical Center, The Netherlands, of heart disease patients found that those who were taking medication for their accompanying depression benefited from even a low dosage of 400 mg per day of EPA and DHA over forty months (Giltay, 2011).

Also in 2011, a meta-analysis of the effects of EPA in clinical trials in depression was published in the *Journal of Clinical Psychiatry* by Dr. E. Sublette of the New York State Psychiatric Institute and her colleagues. The researchers examined fifteen clinical trials involving 916 participants. Their analysis of the studies evaluated suggest—as had two earlier review studies—that EPA is the effective PUFA component in the treatment of depression (Sublette, 2011). This finding is in contrast to the fact that DHA is the major brain omega-3 PUFA and also is in low levels in the brains of depressed patients in postmortem studies (McNamara, 2007). The researchers will be testing this observation in future clinical trials.

In a commentary published in the same issue of the *Journal of Clinical Psychiatry*, Dr. D. Mischoulon of the Massachusetts General Hospital Depression Clinical and Research Program pointed out that "EPA may have benefits for the overall constellation of symptoms known as MDD [major depression disorder] that exceed those of DHA. On the other hand, DHA may impact the mechanism(s) in the brain that regulate suicidal behavior, independent of MDD status" (Mischoulon, 2011).

In 2012 researchers in Taipei, Taiwan, concluded that omega-3 PUFA concentrations are positively associated with cognitive function, particularly immediate recall, in older people with previous depression. Lower concentrations of omega-3 PUFAs or ALA in red blood cell membranes may be good predictors for cognitive impairment in older people with previous recurrent depression (Chiu, 2012).

LIFT YOUR DEPRESSION

The information in this chapter is intended to help people having depressed moods or mild depression. If you are feeling depressed for more than two weeks, you should seek medical assistance promptly. As we stated earlier, there is no good reason for allowing a temporary depressed mood to develop into a major depression. EPA/DHA supplements will help normal, healthy people with temporary mood problems and most individuals with unipolar depression. It takes a higher dosage of EPA and DHA to improve brain levels quickly enough, so we recommend at least 2,000 mg per day combined of EPA and DHA over several months. The brain requires twelve weeks for DHA restoration (Freeman, 2006). Bipolar depression and schizophrenia are more serious forms of depression that will also benefit from fish oil. This will be discussed next.

Bipolar Disorders and Schizophrenia

As we briefly mentioned in the preceding chapter, EPA and DHA can be lifesaving for people suffering from major unipolar depression. It can also be a lifesaver for bipolar disorder and schizophrenia sufferers. Our reason for including this chapter on bipolar disorders and schizophrenia is to inform you of the potentials of omega-3, long-chain polyunsaturated fatty acids (LC-PUFAs) and to encourage you to inform any friends or relatives you have who may be suffering from either of these illnesses.

Why do we say that EPA and DHA can be lifesaving for bipolar and schizophrenic patients? The greatest reason is that omega-3 fatty acids can help reduce suicide. Another important reason is that omega-3s can help such patients improve their mental health. A third vital reason is that omega-3s help patients reduce their use of medications, which can have severe side effects including increased risk of suicide. Bipolar disorder is characterized by recurrent manic or hypomanic and depressive episodes. It afflicts 1.5 percent of Americans, and increases the risk of suicide five- to seventeenfold relative to the general population. Schizophrenia affects an estimated 2.2 million Americans each year, and increases the risk of suicide fiftyfold relative to the general population.

There are 765,000 reported suicide attempts each year in the United States, with about 30,000 of these attempts successful. That equates to eighty-four suicides a day or one every seventeen minutes. A 2004 study examined blood samples of 100 suicide-attempt patients and compared the blood samples to those of 100 mentally healthy controls and found that levels of EPA were significantly lower in the red blood cells of the suicide-attempt patients (Huan, 2004). These findings suggest that low levels of omega-3 LC-PUFAs in tissues may be a risk factor of suicide attempt. Various studies are investigating this link, including one being conducted by the U.S. military (see inset below).

SELF-INFLICTED CASUALTIES OF WAR

Suicides among our servicemen and -women are at an unacceptable level. Between 2005 and 2009, 1,100 servicemen and -women committed suicide, which represents one suicide every day and a half, according to a report from

the Defense Health Board. During that time the Army's suicide rate doubled. According to findings published in the *Journal of Clinical Psychiatry,* male U.S. military personnel on active duty between 2002 and 2008 with the lowest levels of DHA were at a 62 percent increased risk of suicide than counterparts with higher levels. The researchers analyzed data from 800 U.S. military suicide deaths and compared this with 800 control subjects. Results showed, in spite of the fact that this U.S. military population had a very low and narrow range of EPA and DHA, that for every incremental decrease in DHA levels, the risk of suicide death increased by 14 percent. In addition, the risk was significant among men, with the lowest DHA levels associated with a 52 percent increase in suicide risk (Lewis, 2011).

The U.S. military began a study in January 2011 with around 250 service members from three U.S. bases in Iraq, who had served for various lengths of time and performed a variety of functions from infantry to aviation. Although the results are not known at this writing, the study's director, Dr. D. Johnston, Army lieutenant colonel and brigade surgeon for the Enhanced Combat Aviation Brigade deployed in Iraq, suggests that fish oil will reduce this unacceptable rate of suicide and save hundreds of military lives. The study aims to determine whether taking fish oil daily (2.52 grams) for eight weeks will improve soldiers' moods and perceived stress compared with a placebo treatment of omega-6 corn oil. Blood levels of EPA will be tested at the start of the trial and at its close. The effects of the capsules will be measured by a set of psychological tests, and the data will be compared to the results of a placebo drug. Johnston's hypothesis is that soldiers taking the omega-3 supplements will exhibit higher cognitive performance, better mood state, and fewer combat symptoms (Hale, 2010).

"Depending on the results of this research and future research," Johnston stated, "Omega-3 EPA/DHA may be a candidate for a type of 'immunization approach' for depression and other mood disorders when a soldier deploys to an omega-3 deficient and mentally and emotionally strenuous environment." He also noted that in addition to suicide prevention, supplementing soldiers' diets with omega-3s may speed recovery from traumatic brain injury and improve the cockpit skills of aircrew. Stress-related disorders are among the most prevalent and expensive medical consequences of participation in military operations, according to Johnston. Based on his theory, we would certainly recommend fish oil supplements for all servicemen and -women.

BIPOLAR MOOD DISORDERS

Unipolar mood disorders differ from bipolar mood disorders in that there is no associated mania, or high mood. This is just another way of saying that there are two extremes of mood with bipolar disorder, with one extreme being depression and the other an extremely heightened or elevated mood. In the lay sense, mania is the opposite of depression. A person oscillates between one extreme and the other, alternating periods of melancholy and mania.

There is no clear consensus as to how many types of bipolar disorder exist. Bipolar disorder is considered to be a spectrum of disorders by many psychiatrists, who have found that there are at three specific subtypes and one that is non-specified:

1. Bipolar I disorder involves one or more manic episodes; a depressive or hypomanic episode is not required for diagnosis, but it frequently occurs.

2. Bipolar II disorder does not involve a manic episode, but one or more hypomanic episodes and one or more major depressive episode; however, a bipolar II diagnosis is not a guarantee that there will not eventually be such a manic episode in the future.

3. Cyclothymia, a third type, involves a history of hypomanic episodes with periods of depression that do not meet criteria for major depressive

episodes; there is a low-grade cycling of mood which appears to the observer as a personality trait and interferes with functioning.

4. Bipolar disorder NOS (Not Otherwise Specified) is a category that includes all other subtypes of bipolar disorders.

Encouraging Clinical Findings

Here are some studies that illustrate the body of science for EPA and DHA and bipolar disorder. Although the causes and biochemical actions of bipolar disorder are not agreed on, there is evidence that low levels of omega-3 LC-PUFAs are involved and that EPA/DHA supplementation may have a beneficial effect in mitigating symptoms.

- Reduced concentrations of EPA and DHA were reported in red blood cells from bipolar disorder patients under treatment. Investigators analyzed fatty acid levels in twenty bipolar manic patients and twenty healthy controls and found significantly reduced DHA levels in bipolar patients as compared to normal controls (Chiu, 2003).

- Increased rates of bipolar disorder were correlated with reduced intake of seafood containing EPA and DHA. Using data on fish consumption and bipolar disorder incidence, the researchers found that higher seafood consumption indicated a 33 percent lower prevalence of bipolar spectrum disorders, 48 percent lower bipolar I disorder, and 30 percent lower bipolar II disorder (Noaghiul, 2003).

- In two preliminary studies, supplementation with 9.6 grams of EPA and DHA per day, and 1–2 grams per day, respectively, was found to ameliorate bipolar disorder symptoms in two preliminary studies (Stoll, 1999; Frangou, 2006).

- A small clinical study found that eighteen children with juvenile bipolar disorder who were given supplements containing 360 mg per day of EPA and 1,560 mg of DHA for six weeks showed significantly lower levels of both mania and depression, and significantly higher overall functioning after supplementation (Clayton, 2010).

Perhaps these studies are sufficient to encourage you to inform anyone you may know with bipolar disorder to discuss the findings with his or her psychiatrist. Now let's discuss schizophrenia and the therapeutic benefits of EPA and DHA.

SCHIZOPHRENIA

Schizophrenia is a mental disorder in which there is disintegration of thought processes and of emotional responsiveness. It typically manifests in people in their teens and early twenties and usually involves auditory hallucinations, paranoid or bizarre delusions, or convoluted thinking. As associate editor M. Tartakovsky explains so well on PsychCentral.com, "Schizophrenia isn't a split personality: it literally means 'split mind.' Schizophrenia is a chronic, debilitating disorder, characterized by an inability to distinguish between what is real and what isn't. A person with schizophrenia experiences hallucinations and delusional thoughts and is unable to think rationally, communicate properly, make decisions or remember information. To the public, a sufferer's behavior might seem odd or outrageous. Not surprisingly, the disorder can ruin relationships and negatively affect work, school, and everyday activities" (Tartakovsky, 2012).

Schizophrenia has long been considered the most chronic, debilitating, and costly mental illness. Although schizophrenia affects 1 percent of the population, it accounts for a fourth of all mental health costs and takes up one in three psychiatric hospital beds. Since most schizophrenia patients are never able to work, they must be supported for life by Medicaid and other forms of public assistance. The Analysis Group, an economic consulting firm, estimates that the overall U.S. 2002 cost of schizophrenia was $62.7 billion, with $22.8 billion for excess direct health care costs ($7.0 billion outpatient, $5.0 billion drugs, $2.8 billion inpatient, $8.0 billion long-term care). The total direct non-health care excess costs, including living cost offsets, were estimated to be $7.6 billion. The total indirect excess costs were estimated to be $32.4 billion (Wu, 2005).

The American Psychiatric Association's *Diagnostic and Statistical Manual of Mental Disorders* (DSM, fourth edition) is a guideline for classifying the various subtypes of schizophrenia. The DSM lists five subtypes of schizophrenia, although there are regular changes in the number used by various psychiatrists:

1. Paranoid type: Delusions or auditory hallucinations are present, but thought disorder, disorganized behavior, or affective flattening are not. Delusions are persecutory and/or grandiose, but in addition to these, other themes such as jealousy, religiosity, or somatization may also be present.

2. Disorganized type: Where thought disorder and flat affect are present together.

3. Catatonic type: The person may be almost immobile or exhibit agitated purposeless movement. Symptoms can include catatonic stupor and waxy flexibility (a tendency to remain in an immobile posture or position until moved).

4. Undifferentiated type: Psychotic symptoms are present, but the criteria for paranoid, disorganized, or catatonic types are not met.

5. Residual type: This subclassification is diagnosed when a person no longer exhibits symptoms or these symptoms aren't as severe.

Promising Complementary Benefits

Antipsychotic medicines are the cornerstone of schizophrenia treatment but are usually only partially able to alleviate the symptoms. Here's a brief look at several studies that indicate a role for EPA and DHA in the prevention and treatment of schizophrenia.

- A 2001 Dutch study conducted in the Department of Adolescent Psychiatry, University of Amsterdam Medical Center, The Netherlands, found that EPA and DHA were significantly low in nineteen young consecutively admitted schizophrenic patients. The most distinctive findings were that DHA and the total amount of all omega-3 PUFAs were significantly decreased in the patients (Assies, 2001).

- In India, researchers at the National Chemical Laboratory and Interactive Research School for Health Affairs found that levels of EPA and DHA were significantly lower in schizophrenic patients (Ranjekar, 2003).

- A 2010 study from Austria found that EPA and DHA could help delay or prevent the onset of schizophrenia. The researchers enlisted eighty-one high-risk young people, ages thirteen to twenty-four, who had previously suffered brief hallucinations or delusions, and gave half of them capsules of fish oil containing 1.2 grams of EPA and DHA per day, while the other half received a fish-tasting dummy substitute. One year later, only 3 percent of those taking the fish oil capsules had developed schizophrenia compared to 28 percent of those on the substitute. The EPA and DHA were found to prevent the patients from transitioning from a subthreshold psychotic state to a psychotic disorder during the twelve-month study (Amminger, 2010).

- A 2002 South African clinical study using EPA supplements to treat schizophrenia found a positive benefit. The study was a randomized, double-blind, placebo-controlled study conducted over twelve weeks. In the study, forty patients with persistent symptoms after at least six months of stable antipsychotic treatment received three 500 milligrams (mg) of EPA capsules twice daily (3 grams total daily) or a placebo, in addition to their existing treatment. After twelve weeks, the EPA group had significantly greater improvement than the placebo group as measured by Positive and Negative Syndrome Scale (PANSS), a standard medical scale used for measuring symptom severity of patients with schizophrenia. The researchers concluded, "EPA may be an effective and well-tolerated add-on treatment in schizophrenia" (Emsley, 2002).

- Two clinical studies conducted at Sheffield University in the United Kingdom showed improved treatment with fish oil. The first study was designed to distinguish between the possible effects of either EPA or DHA. Forty-five schizophrenic patients on stable antipsychotic medication who were still symptomatic were treated with EPA, DHA, or a placebo for three months. Improvement in those taking the EPA measured by the PANSS was statistically superior to both DHA and the placebo based on changes in percentage scores. EPA was significantly superior to DHA for positive symptoms (hallucinations and delusions) based on follow-up repeated measures.

In the second placebo-controlled study, EPA was used as the sole treatment, though the use of antipsychotic drugs was still permitted if this was clinically imperative. By the end of the study, all twelve patients on the placebo, but only eight out of fourteen patients on the EPA, were taking antipsychotic drugs. Despite this, patients taking EPA had significantly lower scores on the rating scale by the end of the study. The researchers concluded, "EPA may represent a new treatment approach to schizophrenia" (Peet, 2001).

These findings and increasing evidence not only of EPA and DHA's important biological functions in the central nervous system, but also of their importance in treating schizophrenia, led the researchers to explore the existing literature several years later. In 2005 they published a review showing a consistent association between reduced levels of EPA and DHA in cell levels of schizophrenia sufferers that had been found in epidemiological studies. Also, five of six double-blind, placebo-controlled trials reported therapeutic benefit from omega-3 fatty acids, particularly when EPA is added to existing psychotropic medication. The review confirmed that "The evidence to date supports the adjunctive use of omega-3 fatty acids in the management of treatment unresponsive depression and schizophrenia" (Peet, 2005).

• Another clinical trial also reported positive results with fish oil in patients suffering from schizophrenia. Participants in the study, led by Dr. D. Mischuolon at the Massachusetts General Hospital Depression Clinical and Research Program, were previously taking antipsychotic prescription drugs, which after some time were no longer effective After taking EPA, participants in the study experienced progress compared to others who were given a placebo. From January 2003 to June 2006, fifty-seven adults were randomly assigned 1 gram per day of EPA or a placebo for eight weeks in a double-blind, randomized, controlled pilot study. Response criteria were evaluated based on the Depression Rating Scale. EPA demonstrated an advantage over the placebo; however, the low number of patients in the clinical trial prevented the results from reaching statistical significance (Mischoulon, 2009).

- A review by researchers at the Temple University School of Pharmacy on the effects of EPA and DHA in treatment of schizophrenia summarized the literature related to the mechanistic connection between essential fatty acids and schizophrenia and the clinical trials testing fatty acids in patients with schizophrenia. The review found that fatty acids play critical roles in cell membranes of neurons, and certain fatty acids appear to be abnormally low in brains of patients with schizophrenia. The attempt to enhance endogenous (inside the body) levels thus seems a rational and worthwhile goal (Akter, 2011).

The value of such interventions awaits the results of ongoing trials. Despite the limited evidence that supplements ameliorate symptoms of schizophrenia, given the low risk of harm, clinicians might opt to add omega-3 LC-PUFAs to current drug regimens in the hope of better symptomatic control of schizophrenia.

STICKING WITH TREATMENT—AND EPA AND DHA

People with bipolar disorder or schizophrenia should stay on their medication or they probably won't get better. If EPA and DHA merely lowered the need for medication that in itself would be an enormous help and would save countless lives. Fortunately, EPA and DHA do more than lower the need for medication; they positively improve normal brain function. While EPA and DHA supplements are not intended to replace appropriate medication and professional treatment, they do provide additional benefit to existing medicines and also reduce the amount of medication needed, thereby making taking them more tolerable. Most people require two or more medications concurrently to stabilize their mood. Such combinations increase the incidence of serious side effects and often cause patients to stop taking their medications. Omega-3 LC-PUFAs do not have such deleterious side effects, nor do they interact with other medications to increase deleterious side effects. In fact, the primary "side effect" of EPA/DHA supplementation is lower risk of heart disease, which is a bearable cost!

A broad range of dosages of EPA and/or DHA were used in the studies we cite on bipolar disorders and schizophrenia, which makes recommending an optimal dosage difficult. On average, we recommend 1,000–2,000 mg per day, as used in the majority of the positive studies. Keep in mind that this is an active field of research, and by the time you read this book, many more articles will have been published. Much more remains to be known about the potential effects of EPA and DHA on serious mood disorders.

15

Vision

Dietary changes often affect the eye and vision. One of the most well-known examples is vitamin A deficiency, which causes night blindness and complete blindness if the deficiency is severe and long lasting. Reducing the amounts of antioxidants in the diet (found primarily in fresh fruits and vegetables) increases the risk of cataracts. Twenty or so years ago when people were advised to reduce the amount of egg yolk in their diets due to their cholesterol content, a good dietary source of the carotenoids lutein and zeaxanthin needed for the eye's macula was reduced and now there is an increase in age-related macular degeneration. Will the low-fat and no-fat diet fads of the past decades result in retina problems due to decreased intake of EPA and DHA? Can these omega-3 long-chain polyunsaturated fatty acids (LC-PUFAs) slow the loss of vision from these conditions? Let's find out.

CRITICAL NUTRIENTS FOR THE EYE

Vision would not be possible without the presence of EPA and especially DHA. The growing fetus and infant need adequate DHA for eye and brain development. In Chapter 10 on the brain, we mentioned that the retina, a light-sensitive membrane connected to the brain by the optic nerve, has the largest concentration of DHA percentage-wise in the body. DHA is found at high concentrations of 50–60 percent in the retina. It is used by the photoreceptor cells (mainly rods and cones), of which the retina is primarily composed. Photoreceptor cells are responsible for generating electrical signals when stimulated by light, which are then relayed to various areas in the retina that process and organize this information into an image before it is transmitted along the optic nerve fiber to the brain, which interprets the image. Photoreceptor cells are among the most metabolically active in the body, and as such they are critically dependent on essential nutrients for proper eye function.

In the DHA Intake and Measurement of Neural Development (Diamond) Study, a double-blind, randomized, controlled clinical trial of the maturation of infant visual acuity as a function of the dietary level of DHA, researchers examined the effect of four different amounts of DHA supplementation on the visual acuity of formula-fed infants at twelve months of age. The different formulas contained 0 percent, 0.32 percent, 0.64 percent, or 0.96 percent DHA of the fatty acids in the mother's milk substitutes. Infants fed the control formula without DHA had significantly

poorer visual potential and visual acuity at twelve months of age than did infants who received any of the DHA-supplemented formulas (Birch, 2010).

Studies show that no matter one's age omega-3 deficiencies in the diet can lead to long-standing problems with vision. In a study in rhesus monkeys, long-term dietary omega-3 deficiency was associated with two changes in retinal function: a delay in rod recovery that remained relatively constant throughout life; and an age-dependent loss in rod phototransduction sensitivity. In the latter, a lack of dietary carotenoids may have contributed to this decline (Jeffrey, 2009). Both changes affect the complex process that enables us to see.

AGE-RELATED MACULAR DEGENERATION

Age-related macular degeneration (AMD) is the leading cause of severe visual loss in the United States in people over fifty-five, and the leading cause of blindness worldwide. It occurs when the area at the back of the retina called the *macula* begins to degenerate. The macula is an oval, yellow-pigmented area in the center of the retina, containing color-sensitive rods and the central point of sharpest vision. The yellow-pigments are mostly from the dietary carotenoids lutein and zeaxanthin. The National Eye Institute estimated in 2011 that 9 million Americans have AMD. It is also estimated that in the next twenty years, AMD will increase by 50 percent.

The beginning of AMD development may involve ultraviolet destruction of the carotenoid pigments and may have a primary inflammatory component (Penfold, 2001; Donoso, 2006). There are two forms of AMD: dry and wet. In the dry form, or non-neovascular AMD, photoreceptor cells within the macula die off slowly, leaving a pale area in the central part of the eye. In the wet form, or neovascular AMD, abnormal blood vessels grow underneath the macula. These vessels leak blood or fluid, which eventually causes the normal macular tissue to be replaced by scar tissue. Although the dry form is more common than the wet form, with about 85 to 95 percent of people with AMD diagnosed with the dry type, both forms of AMD result in a progressive loss of vision.

In both wet and dry AMD, the disease progresses in stages from early AMD (before there is some noticeable loss of vision) to intermediate AMD (after there is some loss of vision) to advanced AMD (after there is appreciable loss of vision).

Slow Progression of Dry Macular Degeneration

A study at the Australian National University with 33,654 adults, forty-nine years of age or older, found that more frequent consumption of the types of fish that are rich sources of omega-3 LC-PUFAs appears to protect against AMD (Smith, 2000).

The body of scientific evidence suggests that DHA slows vision loss from AMD and other causes. A 2008 review by Dr. T. Cakiner-Egilmez of the Massachusetts Eye and Ear Infirmary in Boston reported that "Studies have also shown that omega-3 fatty acids may slow the progression of vision loss from AMD and reverse the signs of dry eye syndrome" (Cakiner-Egilmez, 2008). (More on dry eye syndrome later.)

A clinical study in 2003 by Dr. J. M. Seddon, also of the Massachusetts Eye and Ear Infirmary, found that a high intake of fish is associated with a lower risk of AMD progression among people with low omega-6 intakes. Processed baked goods, which are abundant in omega-6 fats, increased the rate of AMD progression approximately twofold. The researchers concluded, "Among individuals with the early or intermediate stages of AMD, total and specific types of fat intake, as well as some fat-containing food groups, modified the risk of progression to advanced AMD. Fish intake and nuts reduced risk" (Seddon, 2003).

Seddon and her colleagues followed this study with a 2006 clinical trial known as the U.S. Twin Study of Age-Related Macular Degeneration published in the *Archives of Ophthalmology*. The researchers evaluated AMD risk factors among 681 elderly male twins enrolled in the National Research Council World War II Veteran Twin Registry. Of the participants, 222 were found to have intermediate or advanced AMD.

The results showed that current smokers had a 1.9-fold increased risk of having AMD, while past smokers had a 1.7 increase compared to those who never smoked. (Smoking is high on the list of risk factors for AMD.) For men whose omega-3 intake was among the top 25 percent of participants, there was a 45 percent reduced risk of AMD compared with those whose intake was lower. Eating fish at least twice per week reduced AMD risk by 36 percent compared to those who consumed less than one serving per week. "About a third of the risk of AMD in this Twin Study cohort could be attributable to cigarette smoking, and about a fifth of the cases were estimated as preventable with higher fish and omega-3 fatty acid dietary intake," the researchers concluded (Seddon, 2006).

Another study published in the same issue of the *Archives of Ophthalmology*, this one by Dr. B. Chua and colleagues, also found a decreased risk of developing AMD associated with an increased intake of fish and omega-3 fatty acids. In this Australian study, the researchers analyzed dietary data between 1992 and 1994 from 3,654 men and women, forty-nine years and older, who were enrolled in the Blue Mountains Eye Study. Participants whose omega-3 PUFA intake placed them in the top fifth (20 percent) of subjects were 59 percent less likely to develop early AMD than those whose intake was in the lowest fifth.

Those who consumed fish at least once per week had a similar reduction in early AMD, while those who ate fish at least three times per week had a 75 percent reduction in advanced AMD. As the researchers concluded, "A regular diet high in ω-3 [omega-3] polyunsaturated fat, especially from fish, suggests protection against early and advanced AMD in this older Australian cohort" (Chua, 2006).

Slow Progression of Wet Macular Degeneration

In 2007 Seddon and colleagues in the National Eye Institute Age-Related Eye Disease Study (AREDS) published their findings. In this study, AREDS participants, involving 4,519 sixty- to eighty-year-olds, provided estimates of habitual nutrient intake through a self-reported food-frequency questionnaire. Participants were categorized into four AMD severity groups and a control group. The AREDS researchers found that those who reported the highest dietary intake of omega-3 LC-PUFAs were 39 percent less likely to develop wet AMD compared to those who had the lowest intake. Additionally, those with the highest intake of DHA were 46 percent less likely to develop wet AMD, and those who consumed the most fish (both total and broiled or baked) were 39 percent less likely to develop this condition. In contrast, participants with the highest intake of omega-6 arachidonic acid (AA) were 54 percent more likely to develop wet AMD. The AREDS researchers concluded, "A higher intake of omega-3 LC-PUFAs and fish was associated with decreased likelihood of having NV [wet] AMD" (Seddon, 2007).

In a large European study published in 2008, researchers used food-frequency questionnaires to compare the dietary habits of 105 participants, sixty-five years old, with wet AMD to 2,170 healthy controls. Participants who ate oily fish at least once per week had a 50 percent reduction in the risk of developing wet AMD compared with those who ate fish less than once per week (Augood, 2008).

Decrease Risk of Developing Macular Degeneration

In 2009 researchers at the National Eye Institute reported on their investigation of whether omega-3 LC-PUFA intake was associated with a reduced likelihood of developing wet AMD and central geographic atrophy (CGA) of the retina. CGA is an eye condition associated with advanced dry AMD that involves gradual degradation of retinal cells that can also cause severe vision loss. They found that people who reported the highest omega-3 LC-PUFA intake were 30 percent less likely than their peers to develop wet AMD and CGA. The researchers concluded, "The twelve-year incidence of CGA and NV AMD in participants at moderate-to-high risk of these outcomes was lowest for those reporting the highest consumption of omega-3 LC-PUFAs" (SanGiovanni, 2009).

Also, an earlier study of 4,519 participants by the same AREDS group found that those who reported the highest levels of omega-3 LC-PUFAs in their diet were 30 percent less likely than their peers to develop AMD. They were also 56 percent less likely to progress from bilateral drusen (an eye condition resulting from small accumulations of tissue deposits that displace photoreceptor cells underneath the retina) to CGA. The researchers concluded, "Dietary lipid intake is a modifiable factor that may influence the likelihood of developing sight-threatening forms of AMD. Our findings suggest that dietary omega-3 [LC-PUFAs] is associated with a decreased risk of progression from bilateral drusen to CGA" (SanGiovanni, 2008).

In a study published in 2011, a food-frequency questionnaire was administered at the start of the trial to 39,876 women, ages fifty-four and older. A total of 38,022 women completed the questionnaire and were initially free of AMD. The main outcome measure was incident AMD (the number of women who developed AMD during the study) responsible for a reduction in visual acuity to 20/30 or worse based on a self-report confirmed by a medical record review. A total of 235 cases of AMD were confirmed during an average of ten years of follow-up. Women who were in the highest third of intake for DHA compared with those in the lowest third of intake had a 38 percent lower risk of developing AMD. For EPA, women in the highest third of intake had a 34 percent reduction in risk. Consistent with the findings for DHA and EPA, women who consumed one or more servings of fish per week, compared with those who consumed less than one serving per month, had a 42 percent reduced risk of AMD. The researchers concluded, "These prospective data from a large cohort of female health professionals without a diagnosis of AMD at baseline indicate that regular consumption of DHA and EPA and fish was associated with a significantly decreased risk of AMD and may be of benefit in primary prevention of AMD" (Christen, 2011).

Also in 2011, a French study found similar results. The Alienor Study is a population-based epidemiologic study on nutrition and age-related eye diseases performed in residents of Bordeaux, seventy-three years of age and older. Six hundred sixty-six subjects (that's 1,332 eyes!) with complete data were included in the analyses. The researchers found that subjects with a high intake of omega-3 LC-PUFAs showed a 17 percent decrease in early AMD and a 74 percent decrease in advanced AMD. Associations with advanced AMD were in the same direction (a 26 percent decrease) but did not reach statistical significance. Overall, high intakes of omega-3 LC-PUFAs were associated with 41 percent reduced risk for advanced AMD. The researchers concluded, "These results confirm a decreased risk for AMD in subjects with high intake of omega-3 LC-PUFAs" (Merle, 2011).

DRY EYE SYNDROME

Dry eye (dry eye syndrome, or DES) is a common complaint that is often difficult to treat. According to the National Eye Institute, nearly 5 million Americans, fifty years of age and older, are estimated to have dry eye. Of these, more than 3 million are women and more than 1.5 million are men. Dry eye syndrome is one of the most common causes that bring patients to eye clinics. Tens of millions more have less severe symptoms. DES occurs when the tear glands and the so-called meibomian glands in the eyelid do not produce enough fluid (tears) to keep the eyes moist, resulting in burning and irritation. If the condition becomes severe, it can produce complications leading to eye damage.

There are two major types of dry eye: aqueous tear-deficient dry eye, a disorder in which the lacrimal glands fail to produce enough of the watery component of tears to maintain a healthy eye surface; and evaporative dry eye, a disorder that may result from inflammation of the meibomian glands, also located in the eyelids. Lacrimal and meibomian glands make the lipid or oily part of tears that slows evaporation and keeps the tears stable. Evaporative dry eye is characterized by decreased tear production due to the inflammation. Supplementation with omega-3 fatty acids can reduce the inflammatory compound human leukocyte antigen-DR (HLA-DR) in the thin surface layer of the cornea in individuals with DES.

Resolvin E1, as previously mentioned, is derived from EPA and is involved in inflammation resolution and tissue protection. In an experimental study in mice, resolvin E1 promoted tear production and health, and function of the thin surface layer of the cornea, and decreased inflammatory reactions in the eye. These results suggest that resolvin E1 and similar resolving-like compounds made from EPA and DHA have therapeutic potential in the treatment of DES (Li, 2010).

A review of the body of science regarding dry eye and omega-3 LC-PUFAs was published by Dr. M. Roncone and his Ashton University colleagues in England. In the review summarizing their findings, they wrote, "Evidence suggests that supplementation with omega-3 EFA [essential fatty acids] may be beneficial in the treatment and prevention of dry eye syndrome" (Roncone, 2010).

Another review, this one in 2011 by Drs. A. L. Rand and P. A. Asbell of the Mount Sinai School of Medicine in New York, reported similar results. After their review of the medical literature, they concluded that EPA and DHA appear to be effective against the symptoms of dry eye that many patients experience and that this efficacy is related to their anti-inflammatory effects that we have already described (Rand, 2011).

In 2011 a clinical trial of omega-3 supplements found that the average tear production and tear volume was increased in the omega-3 group as indicated by two diagnostic measuring tools. Patients with dry eye received a daily dose of fish oil, containing 450 milligrams (mg) of EPA, 300 mg of DHA, plus 1,000 mg of flaxseed oil, for three months. As a result, 70 percent of those patients became asymptomatic, whereas for the placebo group, only 7 percent of symptomatic patients became asymptomatic (Wojtowicz, 2011).

Also in 2011, researchers who conducted a study using both omega-3 and omega-6 PUFAs at Paris Descartes University in France concluded, "Supplementation with omega-3 and omega-6 fatty acids can reduce expression [the amount produced] of conjunctival inflammatory markers and may help improve DES symptoms" (Brignole, 2011).

PROTECT YOUR VISION

Well, we hope this discussion has answered some of the questions we posed at the beginning of the chapter. Based on the latest published studies, an intake of 500–1,000 mg per day of EPA and DHA seems to confer protection of the two major eye disorders in our society: AMD and DES Now let's move on to aging of the body and more good news.

16

Cell Aging and Longevity

As people age and become more vulnerable to disease, far too many understand far too well the saying that growing old is not for the faint of heart. Our goal is to help you not just to live longer, but to live better longer. We want to help you live longer without becoming "old." Not just to add years to your life, but life to your years. Most people would agree that quality of life is just as important as length of life.

AGING AND DISEASE

Several factors are involved in the aging process, including free radicals and oxidative stress, glycation caused by excessive blood glucose, genetics, and inflammation. As Dr. A. Ahmad of the Karmanos Cancer Institute in Detroit points out, "Emerging evidence clearly suggests that there is a symbiotic relationship between aging, inflammation, and chronic diseases [. . .] however, it is not clear whether aging leads to the induction of inflammatory processes thereby resulting in the development and maintenance of chronic diseases or whether inflammation is the causative factor for inducing both aging and chronic diseases [. . . .] Moreover, the development of chronic diseases [. . .] could also lead to the induction of inflammatory processes and may cause premature aging" (Ahmed, 2009).

The results from a recent study from the University of Sydney in Australia on the effect of total omega-3 polyunsaturated fatty acids (PUFAs) from fish and nut intakes on the risk of dying from an inflammatory disease are promising. For the study involving 2,514 women, forty-nine and older, researchers collected dietary data using a food-frequency questionnaire, and calculated PUFA, fish, and nut intakes. Over the course of fifteen years, women in the top third of omega-3 consumption had a 44 percent reduced risk of dying from an inflammatory disease compared with those in the lowest third of intake (Gopinath, 2011). The remarkable finding suggests that maintaining optimal levels of omega-3 PUFAs can impact your chances of living longer by helping to control inflammation and aging on a cellular level.

By maintaining and restoring proper cell biochemistry, EPA and DHA can help protect you against the life-shortening, age-related diseases like

heart disease and cancer. EPA and DHA can also help protect you against the quality-of-life-robbing diseases like arthritis and depression. As we discussed in Chapter 2, these omega-3 LC-PUFAs help keep every cell membrane healthier and thus help keep every organ healthier. They are vital ingredients in increasing the fluidity of all membranes. The fluidity of a cell membrane makes possible the movement of biochemical and messenger compounds about the membrane that have important cell-regulating functions throughout the body, and the flow of nutrients and harmful cellular waste into and out from the cell. Proper membrane fluidity is required for cell health and disease prevention.

In this chapter, we will discuss how EPA and DHA can help keep your cells not only healthier, but also younger, and thus help keep your entire body biologically younger.

CHANGES ACCOMPANY AGING

Have you noticed that cuts heal slower and muscles get stiffer as you age? This is due to the aging process, which is distinct from disease processes. People can die of disease at an early age while they still have a biologically young body. Children, for example, can have cancer, high blood pressure, arthritis and other diseases or disorders associated with aging. But people become more susceptible to diseases when they have a biologically old body. There is no physical or mental condition that is directly attributed simply to aging. It is not the passage of time that ages us but rather the gradual loss of cell function that deteriorates our bodies into the condition we call "aged."

Cellular Aging

Aging is the process that reduces the number of healthy cells in the body. The most striking factor in the aging process is the body's loss of reserve, or ability to respond, due to the decreasing number of cells in each organ. For example, fasting blood glucose levels in people remain fairly constant throughout life, but glucose tolerance testing shows a loss of response in aging. (A glucose tolerance test measures the reserve capacity of the endocrine system, specifically the pancreas, to respond to the stress of the glucose load used to challenge the system; glucose is the principal source of food for cells.) This is because cells become less sensitive to the effects of insulin (the hormone produced by the pancreas that moves glucose from the bloodstream into the cells) probably due to the loss of insulin receptor sites on the cell membrane wall. The same diminishment, or slowing down, holds true for the recovery mechanisms of all other body systems. Simply stated, the aging process is the body's gradual loss of ability to respond to a challenge to its status quo (homeostasis). The mass of healthy, active cells in each organ declines as a person ages; thus the organ's function is diminished.

Now the question becomes, What causes this loss of healthy cells?

Cells can die off for several reasons, including membrane dysfunction caused by a deficiency of omega-3 PUFAs. Cells undergo a process called *apoptosis* when they become dysfunctional. Apoptosis is a form of programmed cell death, or "cell suicide," that destroys a cell and then stimulates a cell replacement. Yet, it appears that cells can only replicate properly if they have an adequate amount (length) of telomeres, which are DNA fragments that protect the ends of chromosomes from deterioration. Telomeres can be likened to aglets, the plastic tips that bind the ends of shoelaces to keep them from fraying. Telomeres help keep chromosomes intact much like aglets on shoelaces. As cells replicate over time, the telomeres gradually shorten and the chromosomes lose some of their protection. As telomeres become shorter, eventually cells reach the limit of their replicative capacity, no longer divide or function, and die (Campisi, 2005).

The length of the telomere also influences the stability of genetic information within the DNA. As a result, successive copying can shorten telomeres sometimes to the point that functional genes near the telomeres are lost. which can cause cells not to replicate properly and for cell aberrations to occur. This may play a role in cellular senescence and age-related diseases. Shortened telomeres can be extended by the enzyme telomerase, thus keeping both the telomeres and the genes near them functioning, dividing, and growing. A few nutrients, including EPA and DHA, have been shown to stimulate telemerase production or activity. This will be discussed later in the chapter.

Telomeres can also be thought of as being "countdown clocks" that determine how long you'll live. By slowing the countdown, it is thought that people may be able to extend their lifespan and feel younger longer. Studies show that the shorter your telomeres are, the "older" your body is, regardless of your actual age (Armanios, 2009; Bakaysa, 2007; Omer, 2009; Fitzpatrick, 2011). Shorter telomeres are not only associated with poorer health and biological aging, but also, in particular, white blood cell telomere length (considered to be the main infantry of our bodies' defenses) has been shown to predict survival rates among people with cardiovascular disease (Olovnikov, 1996).

HOW EPA AND DHA AFFECT LONGEVITY AND BIOLOGICAL AGE

If the aging process is slowed, people can live longer. But lifespan, as we've said, is only part of the goal. We want increased lifespan and quality of life. We can easily measure longevity and lifespan objectively, but measuring quality of life is more subjective. Quality of life involves many subjective criteria, but one definite criterion is younger biological age. How does one measure biological age? Let's look at how EPA and DHA affect the markers for longevity first, then at those for biological age.

Longevity

EPA and DHA affect both longevity and aging rate because of their critical role in so many biological processes. A 2009 survey found that low-dietary omega-3 intake is responsible for an estimated 84,000 extra deaths per year in the United States (Danaei, 2009). The beneficial effect of EPA and DHA on longevity has been demonstrated by several studies.

Recall the results from the New Zealand Adolescents and Adults study. In that study 2,416 New Zealanders completed self-assessments of their physical and mental well-being and provided blood samples. Researchers found a significant positive trend in physical and mental well-being in people with the highest levels of EPA in their blood (among the top 20 percent) and the lowest levels of arachidonic acid (AA, an omega-6 pro-inflammatory compound); they were in the bottom 20 percent (Crowe, 2007).

Remember too the large study in 2008 that found that higher intakes of EPA and DHA are associated with a reduced risk of dying prematurely from all causes of death, not just heart-related conditions. This study, which intended to investigate the effect of EPA and DHA on atrial fibrillation (a common irregular heart rhythm), found that EPA/DHA levels were associated with an 85 percent reduction in premature deaths from any and all causes (Macchia, 2008).

A similar beneficial effect was reported in the 2010 Heart and Soul Study. This study, which investigated the effect of psychosocial factors on cardiovascular events in 956 people with stable coronary artery disease, found that those with the highest blood levels of EPA and DHA (among the top 25 percent of participants) were 27 percent less likely to die from any cause, not just heart-related conditions (Pottala, 2010).

Other studies have found similar relationships between blood levels of omega-3 LC-PUFAs and your chances of living longer. In a Swedish study, Dr. M. Lindberg recruited 254 frail, elderly, acutely sick patients and measured their dietary intakes of EPA, which was used as a surrogate marker for dietary intake of marine fatty acids. Over the course of three years of follow-up, the researchers found that those with the lowest EPA blood levels were about 40 percent more likely to die, compared to people with higher levels (Lindberg, 2008).

In a Norwegian randomized, placebo-controlled study, researchers gave 563 men between the ages of sixty-four and seventy-six, at high-risk of cardiovascular disease, 2.4 grams of omega-3 PUFAs per day for three years. During that time, the group had a 47 percent reduction in risk of dying from all causes and an 11 percent reduction in risk of dying from cardiovascular events compared with a placebo group (Einvik, 2010).

Enough said! Now, let's look at the biomarkers that can be used to measure biological age and the protective effects of EPA and DHA.

Biological Age

We mentioned that the shortening of telomeres is thought to be a cause of poorer health and aging. The good news is that the body has enzymes called telomerases that help replenish telomeres and maintain proper telomere length in cells. Fish oils, as you just learned, can protect telomeres from shortening. The mechanisms behind this protective effect are unknown, but may be due to the ability of omega-3 PUFAs to help reduce oxidative stress and increase telomerase activity. Oxidative stress, or cell damage by free radicals, is a powerful driver of telomere shortening. Supplementation with omega-3 PUFAs is associated with lower levels of F2-isoprostanes, a marker for measuring systemic oxidative stress, and higher levels of antioxidant enzymes that protect against the formation of free radicals (Romieu, 2008).

Omega-3 PUFAs are also thought to decelerate telomere shortening by helping to up-regulate (increase production by genes) of telomerase. In experiments, EPA and DHA demonstrated a positive effect on telomerase activity (Chan, 2004).

Dr. R. Farzaneh-Far of the University of California, San Francisco and colleagues at several other institutions recently published two articles on EPA and DHA and telomere lengthening based on findings from their cohort study involving 608 heart attack patients recruited from the Heart and Soul Study, briefly mentioned above. For their investigation blood samples drawn at the time of enrollment were measured for levels of EPA and DHA, and cell telomere length was analyzed. After five years of follow-up, individuals whose EPA/DHA levels were among the lowest 25 percent of participants experienced the fastest rate of telomere shortening, whereas those whose levels were in the highest 25 percent experienced the slowest rate of telomere shortening. Each standard deviation increase in DHA/EPA levels was associated with a 32 percent reduction in telomere shortening (Farzaneh-Far, 2010).

Our discussion of biological aging wouldn't be complete if we didn't remind you that omega-3 PUFAs help keep the skin healthier, softer, and younger looking. As we discussed in Chapter 5 on essential fats, the original reseach by Drs. George and Mildred Burr came about as a result of the need for omega-3 PUFAs and healthy skin. Omega-3 PUFAs are critical for radiant, healthy skin cells. Because they reduce the inflammation that can lead to wrinkles, these fatty acids affect how healthy the skin looks and feels. Their roles in skin health are diverse and include maintenance of the stratum corneum (which is the outermost of the five layers of the epidermis and is largely responsible for the vital barrier function of the skin), inhibition of pro-inflammatory eicosanoids, elevation of the sunburn threshold, and inhibition of pro-inflammatory compounds among other actions (McCusker, 2010). EPA and DHA can be thought of as being internal moisturizers as thay improve skin hydration and firmness. Their stabilizing effects and improvements of cellular membranes may be responsible for changes of skin functions related to skin hydration (De Spirt, 2009).

A biologically young body that helps keep you free of disease, with young-looking skin, is an outward sign that inwardly you're as healthy as possible.

IMPACT YOUR CHANCES OF LIVING LONGER AND BETTER

These results are encouraging: fewer deaths, longer lives, and younger bodies! This is not to say that EPA and DHA are miracle nutrients or a fountain of youth—but optimal amounts of omega-3 LC-PUFAs will help many people live better longer and age more slowly than they would if they were deficient in EPA and DHA. While more research is needed to better define what optimal amounts are and how genetics, lifestyle, and other nutrients impact each individual's aging process, a realistic estimate based on the current body of science suggests that 500–1,000 mg of EPA and DHA per day would be a reasonable range of intake for most of us.

Arthritis

Today, fish oil, the largest source of EPA and DHA, is widely known for its protection against heart disease and relief from arthritis. Even before fish (body) oil was known for its relief of arthritis, there were folk medicine stories of cod liver oils relieving the pain of arthritis. What's the connection between protection from heart disease and protection from arthritis? How did the early research move from heart disease to arthritis?

As described in Chapter 1, insight into the protective benefits of omega-3 fatty acids was first observed in the Greenland Inuits. Initially, it was the life and death condition of heart disease—and the Inuits' lack of it—that caught the attention of Dr. Dyerberg and his colleagues, as did their high omega-3 diet. However, it wasn't too many years later that various researchers found that the Inuits also experienced much lower incidences of other diseases plaguing their Westernized brethren. The high-fat diets of the Inuits had often been ridiculed by contemporary Western nutritionists, yet their diet produced healthier people, having less incidence of the diseases associated with aging. Inuits moving to Denmark and adopting a Western diet developed the same diseases as did the Danes and other Westernized peoples. This important observation removed genetic factors as an explanation and isolated dietary factors as being responsible.

Now flash forward thirty years. A recent study in Yup'ik Eskimos that examined EPA/DHA consumption across a broad range of intake found that increasing EPA/DHA intakes is associated with lower indicators of chronic diseases. (Yup'ik Eskimos have a mean intake of EPA and DHA that is twenty times greater than the current mean intake of the average American, but that is their *mean* intake.) Their intakes go across a wider range, and the researchers found that as their intakes increased to very high levels, their health was better. The findings led researchers to conclude that "increasing EPA/ DHA intakes to amounts well above those consumed by the general U.S. population may have strong beneficial effects on chronic disease risk" (Makhoul, 2010). One such chronic disease is arthritis.

THE ARTHRITIS–HEART DISEASE CONNECTION

Heart disease and arthritis seem to be widely different problems, but both involve inflammation. True, blood clots can cause heart attacks and stroke, and as the early studies in the 1970s with the Greenland Inuits

showed, EPA and DHA reduce that risk. But, in addition to dangerous blood clots, heart attacks and stroke are also caused by inflammation. Heart disease is in large part due to an inflammatory process in the arteries; arthritis is due to inflammation in one or more joints. EPA and DHA reduce inflammation.

Those of you who have read Chapter 4 already know that EPA and DHA possess potent anti-inflammatory properties. Some effects of omega-3, long-chain polyunsaturated fatty acids (LC-PUFAs) are brought about by a modulation in the amount and type of anti-inflammatory eicosanoids that are produced. Other effects are elicited by eicosanoid-independent mechanisms, including actions involving cell signaling, gene expression (the activation of information encoded in a gene), and transcription factor (proteins that control the transfer of information from the genes) (Jump, 2008). The link between inflammation and cardiovascular disease has become so well established that that alone is a compelling reason for anyone suffering from arthritis to be sure to consume optimal amounts of EPA and DHA. In people with rheumatoid arthritis, there is an approximately twofold increase risk of dying, due largely to increased cardiovascular disease (Maradit-Kremers, 2005).

While the heart disease–arthritis link was not known when EPA/DHA supplements were first introduced into the Western diet, many discovered that their arthritis symptoms diminished as they began taking fish oil supplements to protect against heart disease. These serendipitous personal observations (so-called studies of one), plus the epidemiological findings that Inuits had less severe arthritis, eventually led to placebo-controlled clinical studies. The prevalence of rheumatoid arthritis (RA) and osteo-arthritis (OA) was not found to be lower in Inuits, but their symptoms were significantly milder (Recht, 1990).

Since then, dozens of clinical studies have demonstrated the bene-fits of EPA/DHA supplementation in treating arthritis. While omega-3 LC-PUFAs cannot cure arthritis, they have been shown to reduce the inflammation that adds to the progression of arthritis, alleviate the symp-toms of pain and stiffness, decrease the needed dosage of analgesics (pain-relievers) and their side effects, and minimize the added risk that arthritis sufferers have in developing heart disease.

In a study in RA patients, those who chose not to take fish oil were compared with patients who were taking fish oil over a three-year period. Remission in RA activity at three years was more frequent with fish oil use (72 percent) compared to no fish oil (31 percent). Researchers further concluded that fish oil intake reduces cardiovascular risk in patients with RA through multiple mechanisms (Cleland, 2006).

MAJOR TYPES OF ARTHRITIS

According to the U.S. Centers for Disease Control and Prevention (CDC), arthritis is the most common cause of disability in the United States, lim-iting the activities of nearly 21 million adults. The word *arthritis* actually means joint inflammation. According to the CDC, the term is used to describe more than 100 rheumatic diseases and conditions that affect the joints, the tissues that surround the joints, and other connective tissue.

Osteoarthritis

The most common form of arthritis is osteoarthritis (OA), also known as degenerative joint disease or wear-and-tear arthritis. It is characterized by degeneration of the joint cartilage, which acts as cushion between bones to prevent them rubbing against each other. The constant friction breaks down these tissues, triggering the inflammation that eventually leads to pain and joint stiffness. The joints most commonly affected are the knees, the hips, and those in the hands and spine.

According to the CDC, OA of the knee is one of five leading causes of disability among adults. About 80 percent of people with OA have some degree of movement limitation and 25 percent cannot perform major activities of daily living; 11 percent of those with knee OA need help with personal care; and 14 percent require help with routine needs. About 40 percent of adults with knee OA reported their health as "poor" or "fair." In 1999 adults with knee OA reported more than thirteen days of lost work due to health problems. According to the CDC, hip/knee OA ranks high in disability-adjusted life years (early death) and years lived with disability.

Overall, OA affects 13.9 percent of adults ages twenty-five and older and 33.6 percent (12.4 million) of those sixty-five and older—an estimated 26.9 million Americans in 2005, up from 21 million in 1990. Incidence rates increase with age and level off around eighty. Women have higher incidence rates than men, especially after age fifty. Men have 45 percent lower incident risk of knee OA and 36 percent reduced risk of hip OA than women. Prevalent knee OA, but not hip or hand OA, is significantly more severe in women compared to men.

The health care costs are considerable. Average medical costs of OA are about $2,600 per year in patient out-of-pocket expenses. The total annual OA cost per person is about $5,700. The total job-related OA costs in the United States is somewhere between $3.4 billion and $13.2 billion per year.

Rheumatoid Arthritis

RA, an autoimmune condition, is a chronic inflammatory polyarthritis, meaning that it manifests in multiple joints of the body. The inflammatory process primarily affects the lining of the joints (synovial membrane), but it can also affect other organs. The inflamed synovium leads to erosions of the cartilage and bone and sometimes to joint deformity. Pain, swelling, and redness are common joint manifestations.

In 2005, using a more restrictive definition than in earlier estimates, the CDC estimated that 1.3 million U.S. adults aged eighteen and older had RA. There is almost a 2:1 ratio in prevalence for women to men, with 1,367 per 100,000 among women compared with 736 per 100,000 in men.

A study of medical costs among people with RA at the Mayo Clinic found an average cost of $3,802.05 per person in the year 1997 (Gabriel, 1997). The study also reported that people with RA were approximately six times more likely than people without arthritis to incur medical charges. These charges were not just for musculoskeletal disorders but also for care of disorders of most body systems. Another study estimated the median lifetime costs (that is, twenty-five years following diagnosis) of RA to be $61,000 to $122,000 (Gabriel, 1999).

Systemic Lupus Erythematosus

A third major form of arthritis is systemic lupus erythematosus (SLE, or lupus). According to the CDC, lupus is an autoimmune disease in which the immune system produces antibodies to cells throughout the body leading to widespread inflammation and tissue damage. Lupus has a variety of clinical manifestations and can affect the joints, skin, brain, lungs, kidneys, and blood vessels. People with lupus may experience fatigue, pain, or swelling in joints, skin rashes, and fevers. According to a 2008 report from the National Arthritis Data Working Group, approximately 250,000 Americans have SLE.

Women have a higher incidence of SLE than men, thereby suggesting a hormonal relationship. The female-to-male ratio peaks at 11:1 during the childbearing years. A correlation between age and incidence of SLE mirrors peak years of female sex hormone production. Onset of SLE is usually after puberty, typically in the twenties and thirties, with 20 percent of all cases diagnosed during the first two decades of life. The prevalence of SLE is highest among women between fourteen and sixty-four. SLE does not have an age predilection in males, although it should be noted that among older adults, the female-to-male ratio falls.

HOW EPA AND DHA HELP TREAT SYMPTOMS OF ARTHRITIS

Over the years, the body of science regarding the beneficial effect of EPA and DHA from fish oil on arthritis has become substantial. These studies show that it is difficult to get enough EPA and DHA from food alone to maximize their benefits when fighting arthritis. However, studies involving adequate dosages of omega-3 LC-PUFAs (ranging from 1.6–7.1 grams per day) are all encouraging. Several reviews of these trials of fish oil in treating RA and other inflammatory joint-pain disorders have been published, and each concluded that there is benefit from fish oil (Volker, 1996; James, 1997; Geusens, 1998; Kremer, 2000; Calder, 2001).

In an editorial commentary discussing the use of fish oil in RA, two prominent rhematology researchers Drs. L. Cleland and M. James of the Royal Adelaide Hospital in Australia concluded that "The findings of benefit from fish oil in rheumatoid arthritis are robust. . . . Dietary fish oil supplements in rheumatoid arthritis have treatment efficacy. . . . Dietary fish oil supplements should now be regarded as part of the standard therapy for rheumatoid arthritis" (Cleland, 2000).

Reduce Reliance on Arthritis Medications

EPA and DHA have been found to reduce the reliance on analgesics such as ibuprofen, aspirin, acetaminophen, and other nonsteroidal anti-inflammatory drugs (NSAIDs). In spite of their pain-relieving effects, these analgesics do not affect long-term progress of the disease, nor do they have a curative effect. Yet they can have significant side effects, including death. Long-term usage of these medications can cause stomach pain, ulcers, and bleeding and substantially increases the risks for more serious problems such as heart failure, heart attack, and kidney failure. The concomitant use of fish oil can lessen the need for analgesics within weeks and allows many people to dispense with a reliance on analgesics within months.

In one double-blind, placebo-controlled, randomized study, ninety-seven patients with RA were randomly assigned to take 2.2 grams of omega-3 fatty acids a day or placebo capsules. After nine months, 39 percent in the omega-3 group were able to reduce their daily NSAID medications by more than 30 percent (Galarraga, 2008).

In a review of fifteen studies involving the use of fish oil as well as standardized NSAID treatment, Cleland and James reported, "In addition to general application as an NSAID-sparing agent in the Rheumatology

Clinic, we have evaluated long-term use of fish oil in a cohort of patients with recent onset RA, who are treated according to a standardized treatment strategy [. . . .] In this cohort, fish oil has been continued long-term by a majority of subjects. As well as being associated with significantly reduced NSAID use and favorable cardiovascular risk profiles compared to those who do not take fish oil, there was better disease suppression with fish oil use" (Cleland, 2006).

In a brief review also in 2006, Cleland and James concluded, "In summary, fish oil is a safe, acceptable alternative to NSAIDs for arthritis. NSAIDs have the advantage of prompt action, but for long-term use, fish oil has clear advantages in terms of less risks and collateral health benefits" (Cleland, 2006).

Relieve Joint Pain and Tenderness

In a 2007 meta-analysis, Drs. R. Goldberg and J. Katz examined the pain-relieving effects of EPA and DHA in patients with RA, joint pain due to inflammatory bowel disease (chronic inflammation of the digestive tract), or dysmenorrhea (menstrual cramps). Supplementation with omega-3 PUFAs for three to four months reduced patient-reported joint pain intensity, minutes of morning stiffness, number of painful and/ or tender joints, and NSAID consumption. They concluded, "Omega-3 PUFAs are an attractive adjunctive treatment for joint pain associated with rheumatoid arthritis, inflammatory bowel disease, and dysmenorrhea" (Goldberg, 2007). In this analysis, eleven of the sixteen studies used a DHA/EPA dose of 2.7 grams per day and patients noted lessening of pain.

In 2008 at a scientific meeting of the Nutrition Society, Dr. P. Calder of the University of Southampton in England reviewed the body of science regarding arthritis and omega-3 LC-PUFAs and the main mechanism by which they work to reduce inflammation. He reported that EPA and DHA inhibit arachidonic acid (AA) from being converted into inflammatory eicosanoids in the body. EPA also gives rise to eicosanoid mediators that are less inflammatory than those produced from AA, and both EPA and DHA give rise to generations of resolvins, protectins, and maresins, which are potent anti-inflammatory and inflammation-resolving compounds. Further, Calder pointed out that in addition to modifying the numbers of the various mediating-compounds present, "Omega-3 PUFAs exert effects on other aspects of immunity relevant to RA as well." He stated, "Fish oil has been shown to slow the development of arthritis in an animal model and to reduce disease severity. Randomized clinical trials have demonstrated a range of clinical benefits in patients with RA that include reducing pain, duration of morning stiffness, and use of non-steroidal anti-inflammatory drugs" (Calder, 2008).

The inflammatory-attenuating effect of EPA and DHA was recently examined in a Finnish study, testing the hypothesis that high blood levels of omega-3 LC-PUFAs are associated with lower levels of C-reactive protein (CRP) in 1,395 healthy middle-aged Finnish men. The study found that omega-3 LC-PUFA levels were inversely associated with CRP, a marker of inflammation in the body (Reinders, 2011).

For a discussion of inflammation and athletic performance, see the inset below.

INFLAMMATION AND ATHLETIC PERFORMANCE

EPA and DHA are important for reducing the pain and swelling of inflammation that occur in athletes. Sports require repetitive motions, strains, and tears that often lead to inflammation. Athletes may want to consider taking fish oil to help reduce and control inflammation, while protecting muscle mass.

EPA and DHA also help produce muscle and reduce muscle loss. One of the reasons that muscle tissue decreases with age is that cellular insulin sensitivity declines and cells can't adequately incorporate amino acids to build or renew proteins. EPA and DHA improve insulin-mediated glucose metabolism in insulin-resistant states. A 2007 study showed that EPA and DHA improved insulin sensitivity and muscle mass. The researchers, led by Dr. C. Thivierge of the Université Laval's Institute of Nutraceuticals and Functional Foods in Quebec, Canada, found that subjects eating a diet rich in omega-3 menhaden fish for five weeks had improved insulin ability to metabolize amino acids. Their study further showed that the EPA and DHA help produce new muscle proteins and enhance muscle recovery. They concluded, "Chronic feeding of menhaden oil provides a novel nutritional means to enhance insulin-sensitive aspects of protein metabolism" (Gingras, 2007).

A 2011 study published in the *American Journal of Clinical Nutrition* investigated the effect of EPA and DHA on the rate of muscle growth. The scientists randomly assigned a group of older adults to receive 4 grams daily of omega-3 or corn oil for eight weeks. They found that corn oil supplementation had no effect on building muscle, but omega-3 was found to increase the rate of muscle buildup. The authors wrote, "Omega-3 fatty acids stimulate muscle protein synthesis in older adults and may be useful for the prevention and treatment of sarcopenia [age-related loss of muscle mass]" (Smith, 2011).

A 2012 study at Brazil's Federal University of Paraná showed that EPA and DHA improved strength-training benefits in older persons. The study investigated the effect of fish oil supplementation and strength training on muscle strength and functional capacity among older women. In the study, forty-five healthy women in their mid-sixties were randomly assigned to three groups. One group performed strength-training exercises only for ninety days. The other two groups performed the same strength-training program and received 2 grams per day of fish oil for ninety days or for 150 days, respectively, with the latter group starting supplementation sixty days before training began. Muscle strength and function were assessed before and after the training period. All the women showed muscle improvement, but the two fish oil groups improved more and also performed better in a particular test. Only those receiving the fish oil supplements showed improvements in electromechanical measures of muscle performance. The researchers concluded, "Strength training increased muscle strength in elderly women. The inclusion of fish oil supplementation caused greater improvements in muscle strength and functional capacity" (Roadacki, 2012).

FOR LONG-TERM ARTHRITIS RELIEF

If you suffer from the pain and stiffness of arthritis, you should consider giving EPA and DHA a test trial at a sufficient dosage for a sufficient amount of time. Determining the proper dose and the amount of time needed for results may require some trial and error. People differ in their ability to respond to omega-3 LC-PUFAs, and arthritis symptoms differ in people, so there are wide variations in both dosage and time needed for results to appear. A major review of clinical studies has shown that typically "The dose needed for anti-inflammatory effect or long-term analgesia [pain-relief] is 3 grams or more daily of EPA plus DHA" (Cleland, 2009).

To determine an effective dosage for yourself, we recommend starting with 2–3 grams of EPA/DHA per day, and gradually increasing that amount to a maximum of 7 grams per day until your symptoms improve. Allow yourself a reasonable trial period of at least two months. In the meantime, you will also be protecting your brain and cardiovascular system.

18

Diabetes

Modern Westernized diets and sedentary lifestyles have created a diabetes epidemic. The Centers for Disease Control and Prevention (CDC) describes diabetes as a disease in which blood glucose levels are above normal. Most of the food we eat is turned into glucose (a sugar) for our bodies to use for energy. The pancreas, an organ that lies near the stomach, makes a hormone called insulin to help glucose get into the cells in our bodies. When someone has diabetes, his or her body either doesn't make enough insulin (type 1 diabetes) or can't use its own insulin as well as it should (type 2 diabetes). This causes sugar to build up in the bloodstream and has other negative effects such as elevating blood lipids and damaging blood vessels—all of which can cause a number of serious health problems.

Diabetes increases the risk of eye disease, heart disease, neuropathy (nerve damage in the limbs and internal organs), and kidney disease. According to the CDC, diabetes is the seventh leading cause of death in the United States. People with diabetes are more likely to suffer from such complications as heart attacks, strokes, high blood pressure, kidney failure, blindness, and amputations of the feet and legs. Diabetes costs $174 billion annually in the United States, including $116 billion in direct medical expenses. In 2011 the CDC estimated that nearly 26 million Americans have diabetes.

Type 2 diabetes, the more common form of the disease, is primarily a disorder of carbohydrate metabolism due to insulin dysfunction (a defect in insulin action or secretion). The high-fat, low-carbohydrate diet of the Greenland Inuits was protective against diabetes. It did not contribute to insulin resistance (the inability of the cells to respond to insulin effectively) or excessive insulin production. Since there isn't an overly generous supply of seal and whale blubber in Western diets (as there is of refined carbohydrates—another contrast to the Inuit diet), the question becomes, Can providing adequate omega-3 long-chain polyunsaturated fatty acids (LC-PUFAs) in Western diets help reduce the epidemic of type 2 diabetes? Can it protect diabetics from heart disease and the other severe circulatory complications associated with this condition?

Let's take a look at the problem of diabetes and the help that EPA and DHA bring.

TYPES OF DIABETES

The three main types of diabetes are type 1 diabetes, formerly called insulin-dependent diabetes mellitus (IDDM) or juvenile-onset diabetes; type 2 diabetes, formerly called non-insulin-dependent diabetes mellitus (NIDDM) or adult-onset diabetes; and gestational diabetes that only pregnant women get.

Type 1 diabetes is an autoimmune disease in which the immune system attacks the insulin-producing beta cells in the pancreas and destroys them. The pancreas then produces little or no insulin, which requires the diabetic to take insulin daily. This disorder, which generally develops in children and young adults (although it can occur at any age), accounts for about 5 percent of all diagnosed cases of diabetes.

Type 2 diabetes results when the body gradually loses its ability to use and produce enough insulin. This disorder typically appears in adults but is increasingly being diagnosed in children and adolescents as maturity-onset diabetes of the young (MODY). It is usually part of a metabolic syndrome that includes excess weight/obesity, insulin resistance, high triglycerides/low high-density lipoprotein (HDL often called "good") cholesterol, and/or high blood pressure. It accounts for about 90 to 95 percent of all diagnosed cases of diabetes.

Gestational diabetes, not treated, can cause problems for mothers and babies. Gestational diabetes develops in 2 to 10 percent of all pregnancies but usually disappears when a pregnancy is over.

Other specific types of diabetes resulting from specific genetic syndromes, surgery, drugs, malnutrition, infections, and other illnesses may account for 1 to 5 percent of all diagnosed cases of diabetes. In this chapter, we'll focus on type 1 and type 2 diabetes.

HOW EPA AND DHA MAY LOWER RISK OF TYPE 1 DIABETES

Surprisingly, a Norwegian study found that the use of cod liver oil, which is a traditional Norwegian supplement, in the first year of life was associated with a significantly lower risk of type 1 diabetes later in life. The study found that "cod liver oil may reduce the risk of type 1 diabetes, perhaps through the anti-inflammatory effects of long-chain ω-3 [omega-3] fatty acids" (Stene, 2003).

Four years later a mechanism to explain this observation was found in a study conducted in children at increased genetic risk for type 1 diabetes. In this study, dietary intake of omega-3 fatty acids was associated with a lower incidence of autoantibodies in the blood that signal the immune system to attack the insulin-producing beta cells in the pancreas. Since type 1 diabetes is caused by autoantibodies destroying the beta-cells in the pancreas, this research indicates that EPA and DHA may help block inflammation by inhibiting the production of inflammatory compounds by macrophages into body tissues, and thus decrease inflammation that leads to type 1 diabetes (Norris, 2007).

HOW EPA AND DHA MAY LOWER RISK OF TYPE 2 DIABETES

The prevalence of type 2 diabetes in the United States continues to rise. In addition to the nearly 26 million Americans with diabetes, the CDC estimates that as many as one in three U.S. adults could have diabetes by 2050 if current trends continue.

Omega-3 LC-PUFAs have been postulated to reduce type 2 diabetes risk, even if the role of these omega-3 fatty acids and fish intake in the development of type 2 diabetes remains unresolved. An example of the positive effects of EPA and DHA on type 2 diabetes risk is the results from a prospective, population-based Chinese cohort study in 51,963 men and 64,193 women in middle-age who were free of type 2 diabetes at the time of enrollment. Dietary information and intake were collected by a food-frequency questionnaire, with additional dietary assessments every two years for a period of eight years. Fish consumption was grouped into four categories: combined fish and shellfish, shellfish, saltwater fish, and freshwater fish. Higher intakes of fish and shellfish and omega-3 LC-PU-FAs were associated with significantly lower risks of diabetes in women, and higher shellfish consumption was associated with lower diabetes risk in men (Villegas, 2011).

More research is needed to clearly delineate a relationship between EPA and DHA and lower risk of developing type 2 diabetes. However, researchers have begun to understand the mechanisms that make omega-3 LC-PUFAs effective against the cluster of metabolic conditions that precede its development.

Help Prevent Inflammation Associated with Obesity

The increasing prevalence of overweight and obesity is a major contributing factor to the epidemic of type 2 diabetes. The World Health Organization (WHO) estimates that more than 1 million deaths annually in Europe can be attributed to diseases related to excess body weight; in the United States, this estimate is 300,000, according to a recent U.S. Surgeon General's report. And with the rising global obesity levels, these death rates are set to drastically increase. Roughly 80 percent of those with type 2 diabetes are overweight.

A report on obesity, inflammation, and diabetes by Drs. E. Oliver and F. McGillicuddy of the University College of Dublin helps to explain how obesity contributes to the development of type 2 diabetes and its precursor insulin resistance: "Obesity is associated with low-grade chronic inflammation characterized by inflamed adipose tissue with increased macrophage infiltration. This inflammation is now widely believed to be the key link between obesity and development of insulin resistance (Oliver, 2010). Insulin resistance can develop when macrophages clustered inside fat tissue secrete a barrage of inflammation-causing chemicals that damage the surrounding cells, rendering them unable to control sugar levels in response to the insulin signal. Thus, the more fatty tissue there is, the more inflammation and the more resistant the cells become to insulin.

Other research by Oliver and McGillicuddy found that activation of pro-inflammatory pathways can "cross talk" with insulin, signaling pathways by a number of mechanisms. They point out that EPA and DHA regulate the expression of genes involved in inflammation through transcription factors such as NF-kappa B, and by increasing anti-inflammatory eicosanoid production and reducing pro-inflammatory cytokine production, as we discussed in Chapter 4. The researchers concluded that EPA and DHA may offer a useful anti-inflammatory strategy to decrease obesity-induced insulin resistance (Oliver, 2010).

Reduce Insulin Resistance

Insulin resistance, also known as prediabetes, often precedes the development of diabetes by many years. It is usually defined on a metabolic level as inefficient insulin function in skeletal muscle, liver, and fat cells. This hampers the normal role of insulin, whereby it causes increased muscle cellular glucose uptake, glycogen synthesis, and cessation of liver glucose production. While all cells can become resistant to insulin, it is the liver cells, muscle cells, and fat cells that carry the major burden of metabolizing glucose. Insulin causes the cells in the liver, muscle, and fat tissue to take up glucose from the blood, storing it as glycogen in the liver and muscle. If needed, the liver can metabolize this stored glycogen into glucose to keep the body glucose levels within normal range. If the muscles and fat cells become resistant to insulin, they cannot burn the glucose the liver makes. If all these major tissues become resistant, the pancreas is forced to put out more insulin to compensate and to attempt to normalize blood glucose levels. Gradually, the pancreas becomes overburdened and can no longer produce enough insulin. When the increased insulin production caused by insulin resistance fades out, blood glucose levels remain permanently high and type 2 diabetes is present.

The following studies with EPA and DHA show that this progression to type 2 diabetes is not inevitable. Working at the cellular level, EPA and DHA help improve the uptake of insulin by the cells and the proper processing of glucose and triglycerides/cholesterol—all conditions, that if working properly, reduce the risk of insulin resistance from developing into type 2 diabetes.

Improve Insulin Activity

Early laboratory animal studies indicated that EPA and DHA have a beneficial effect on insulin sensitivity. Insulin sensitivity is a measure of how well, or how sensitive, the insulin receptor in the cell membrane is to taking glucose into the cell. In 1991 it was determined that high levels of some dietary fats, particularly triglycerides, have a major impact on insulin sensitivity. Appropriate amounts of EPA effectively reduced elevated blood triglycerides. If the effect of triglycerides on insulin sensitivity in animal studies also applies to humans, then fish oil would have a protective effect against diabetes.

In a well-designed animal study, Dr. L. Storlien and colleagues determined that diets high in omega-6 PUFAs or saturated, monounsaturated (omega-9) fats led to severe insulin resistance. Substituting 11 percent of the fatty acids in the animals' omega-6 PUFA diet with EPA and DHA normalized insulin action in the animals. Substituting 11 percent of fatty acids in the PUFA fat diet with omega-3 LC-PUFAs from fish oils normalized insulin action in the animals. Replacing 11 percent of the omega-6 PUFA diet with the shorter-chain omega-3 alpha-linolenic acid (ALA) was ineffective in the PUFA diet in normalizing insulin action in the animals. However, ALA completely prevented the insulin resistance induced by a saturated fat diet. Insulin sensitivity in skeletal muscle was inversely correlated with mean muscle triglyceride accumulation. Furthermore, the percentage of omega-3 LC-PUFAs correlated highly with insulin action in muscles.

This study produced several important findings about the actions of EPA and DHA. One was that insulin sensitivity was inversely correlated with muscle triglyceride accumulation, and the second was that the percentage of EPA and DHA in phospholipid correlated highly with insulin action. From these findings, the researchers concluded that the type of high-fat diet consumed can influence the uptake of insulin by the cells in animals, and that EPA and DHA can lower triglyceride levels as well as have a positive influence on regulating insulin (Storlien 1991).

However, laboratory animal studies are not human clinical trials. Direct experimental testing of these possibilities has been difficult, because omega-3 fatty acids may affect metabolism differently in animals than in humans.

In 2007 it was found that insulin sensitivity improved after twelve weeks of daily supplementation with 1.3 grams of EPA and 2.9 grams of DHA in thirty overweight and obese premenopausal non-diabetic women. Also, the inflammatory markers (C-reactive protein and interleukin-6) were significantly lower after twelve weeks of EPA/DHA supplementation (Browning, 2007).

In that respect a recent study of seventy-six children, nine to eighteen years old, who were overweight and insulin resistant but otherwise healthy, is interesting. The children were randomly assigned to receive either 900 mg of omega-3 LC-PUFAs daily or a placebo for one month. No dietary intervention was conducted. Despite no differences at baseline, only the omega-3 group decreased fasting insulin and insulin resistance assessed by the homeostatic model assessment, which is a method used to quantify insulin resistance. Significant differences between groups were also observed for changes in inflammatory markers (TNF-α, leptin, and adiponectin) after omega-3 supplementation (Lopez-Alarcón, 2011).

Improve Glucose Control

Impaired glucose tolerance (IGT) is a prediabetic state that is associated with insulin resistance. IGT may precede type 2 diabetes mellitus by many years. It is a condition in which blood sugar levels are higher than normal, but not high enough to be diagnosed as diabetes. An estimated 79 million U.S. adults have impaired glucose tolerance.

By 1994 it was known from Finnish and Dutch cohorts of the Seven Countries Study that men who consumed fish two to three times per week or who took an omega-3 supplement were better able to manage their blood glucose levels after a twenty-year follow-up (Feskens, 1994). In 1997 increased fish consumption was associated with reduced risk of developing IGT (Vilbersson, 1997).

Additional epidemiologic support came in 2004. A study of Icelandic men found that their incidence of type 2 diabetes was lower than that of other Nordic men, despite the fact that the Icelandic men were more overweight or obese. Dr. I. Thorsdottir and colleagues determined that the lower incidence of type 2 diabetes in Icelandic men was associated with the higher omega-3 PUFA/EPA content and the lower omega-6 content in the Icelandic milk compared with milk from other Nordic countries (Thorsdottir, 2004).

In a 2005 review of the body of science on this topic published in the *Journal of the American Dietetic Association*, Drs. J. Nettleton and R. Katz remarked that "Historically, epidemiologic studies have reported a lower prevalence of impaired glucose tolerance and type 2 diabetes in populations consuming large amounts of the omega-3 LC-PUFAs found mainly in fish. Controlled clinical studies have shown that consumption of omega-3 LC-PUFAs has cardioprotective effects in persons with type 2 diabetes without adverse effects on glucose control and insulin activity." The evidence also suggested that "Increased consumption of omega-3 LC-PUFAs with reduced intake of saturated fat may reduce the risk of conversion from impaired glucose tolerance to type 2 diabetes in overweight persons" (Nettleton, 2005).

In 2009 a paper published by Dr. M. Vaquero and associates at the Spanish National Research Council in Madrid reviewed the various biochemical pathways in which omega-3 PUFAs improve glucose metabolism and insulin sensitivity. They remarked that an increase in the amount and degree of unsaturation of the muscle membrane fatty acids is associated with improved insulin sensitivity. They suggested that a higher proportion of omega-3 fatty acids in the diet may have beneficial roles, such as anti-obesity effects and protection against the metabolic syndrome and type 2 diabetes mellitus through a number of metabolic effects. Based on these findings, the researchers concluded that "fish oil [. . .] has many physiological effects; indeed, it reduces insulin response to oral glucose without altering the glycemic response in healthy humans" (Martín de Santa Olalla, 2009).

Improve Triglycerides and Unhealthy Cholesterol Levels

The body needs insulin to remove fats from the blood. People with pre-diabetes and diabetes often have high triglyceride levels and low HDL (good) cholesterol levels. EPA and DHA are effective in reducing blood triglycerides and platelet reactivity in diabetics (De Caterina, 2007). The increased risk of coronary artery disease (see following discussion) among people with diabetes is attributable, in part, to specific disorders of lipoprotein metabolism that are common in this population. These include impaired metabolism of very-low-density lipoproteins (VLDL) and/or chylomicrons (very small molecules that transport cholesterol, tri-glycerides, and other fats through the bloodstream) and are thought to play the largest role in irritating the artery walls and causing inflammation that can lead to plaque formation. Elevated triglycerides after food intake have been associated with both early coronary artery disease and carotid artery atherosclerosis. (Fats and oils in food are mostly found in triglyceride form, a chemical form that is more favorable for storing fatty acids compactly in the body and for transporting them in the blood.)

In 2011 a prospective study of 3,088 older adults followed for more than ten years found that individuals with the highest blood levels of EPA and DHA, as well as their precursor ALA, were about 25 percent less likely to develop diabetes than those with the lowest levels (Djoussé, 2011). Also in 2011, researchers, led by Dr. G. Derosa of the University of Pavia in Italy confirmed that omega-3 boosts insulin resistance markers. The researchers determined that increased consumption of omega-3 fatty acids helps to improve important indicators of insulin function. The study evaluated the effects of omega-3 PUFAs on lipid profile and insulin resistance biomarkers. The researchers found that dietary intake of omega-3 capsules with meals resulted in improved lipid profiles and adiponectin (a hormone associated with a greater risk of obesity) levels, compared to the placebo, and an improvement of all insulin resistance parameters after fat-containing meals.

For the study, 167 patients were given 1 gram of either EPA and DHA or a placebo three times a day, during meals, for six months. The EPA/DHA supplement was reported to improve HDL cholesterol and tri-glyceride levels compared to the placebo after a fat-containing meal, while the supplement had a neutral effect on total cholesterol and low-density lipoprotein (LDL or "bad") cholesterol. The researchers found that the group taking the EPA/DHA supplement showed an improvement of all parameters *including indicators of insulin resistance,* while there was no effect with the placebo (Derosa, 2011).

Most, but not all, clinical studies demonstrate that fish, fish oil, or EPA/DHA supplements reduce insulin resistance. Discrepancies in study findings may be due to differences in health status of participants; the macronutrient, fatty acid, and antioxidant nutrient composition of their diet; the amount, duration, and fatty acid composition of the omega-3 PUFAs used in the trials; and the methods used to assess insulin resistance. Using only low amounts of omega-3 PUFAs does not seem to affect glucose control in type 2 diabetics. Greater amounts may be necessary to achieve significant results. As such, people with diabetes or prediabetes should consider EPA/DHA dosages of 1–2 grams per day to improve their insulin sensitivity and 2–4 grams per day to lower high blood triglycerides.

HOW EPA AND DHA HELP DIABETES-RELATED AILMENTS

If not controlled, abnormally high levels of glucose in the blood eventually damage blood vessels, which in turn, can lead to eye disease, heart disease, kidney and liver diseases, and other serious health problems. Let's briefly look at two of the more common diabetes-related ailments—heart disease and liver disease—and whether EPA and DHA can help protect people against them, and if so, how. We'll start with heart disease, as this benefit alone would make EPA and DHA critical to the long-term health of all diabetics and those with prediabetic conditions like insulin resistance.

Heart Disease

A 2002 review of the body of science on this topic by Drs. C. Sirtori and C. Galli of the University of Milan in Italy examined both the effect of omega-3 PUFAs on insulin sensitivity and cardiovascular health. Their review examined large population studies, including their own, and led the researchers to conclude that "while diabetes development was in no way accelerated in any of these studies, there was, instead, clear evidence of a significant hypotriglyceridemic [blood triglyceride-lowering] activity of the supplements. In long-term treatments, there was also a tendency toward a significant reduction of low-density lipoprotein (LDL), with positive effects on high-density lipoprotein (HDL). These findings fit well with cellular changes indicative of improved glucose handling. Finally, recent data suggest an improvement of heart rate variability by fish intake in coronary patients that is also exerted by the omega-3 fatty acids, thus providing further indication for the potential benefit of such treatments in diabetic patients" (Sirtori, 2002).

A similar effect on heart rate is further documented in a U.S. study among 3,326 men and women, sixty-five and older, who were free of irregular heartbeats due to atrial fibrillation or heart failure at the time of their enrollment. Blood levels of EPA and DHA were also measured at the same time. During 31,169 person-years of follow-up from 1992 to 2006, higher (total) omega-3 LC-PUFA and DHA levels were associated with lower risk of atrial fibrillation, and thereby irregular heartbeats (Wu, 2012).

Dr. A. Stirban and colleagues at Ruhr-University Bochum in Germany investigated the effects of EPA and DHA on vascular function that normally occurs after meals in people with type 2 diabetes. The first few hours after eating poses high risks for diabetics, whose blood glucose and insulin levels rise sharply, increasing their risks for cardiovascular events. In their double-blind, placebo-controlled, randomized, crossover study, thirty-four subjects with type 2 diabetes received either 2 grams of EPA and DHA or a placebo daily for six weeks. The investigators evaluated blood flow in the participants at two, four, and six hours following a high-fat meal. They observed that a decrease in dilation of the larger blood vessels (arteries) was significantly less for those who consumed the EPA and DHA compared with those taking the placebo. Additionally, EPA/DHA supplementation improved functioning of smaller blood vessels (capillaries, venules, and arterioles) after meals. These observations suggest a protective vascular effect of EPA and DHA (Stirban, 2010).

At the Lipid Research Center in Quebec, Dr. I. Rudkowska conducted a literature review examining the impact of fish oil supplementation on blood lipids, glycemic control, blood pressure, and inflammation in people with type 2 diabetes. In a discussion of his findings, Rudkowska remarked, "The literature suggests that omega-3 LC-PUFA supplementation presents many benefits in type 2 diabetes management mainly in terms of dyslipidemia [abnormal amounts of lipids and lipoproteins in the blood]. Overall, omega-3 LC-PUFA supplementation represents a reasonable therapeutic strategy in individuals with type 2 diabetes to decrease the risk of complications" (Rudkowska, 2010).

Non-Alcoholic Fatty Liver Disease

The accumulation of fat in the liver is a result of the disordered control of fats that occurs in insulin resistance or diabetes. In non-alcoholic fatty liver disease (NAFLD), which is strongly associated with diabetes and heart disease, triglyceride deposits build up inside the liver, blocking its hundreds of functions. In 2010 Dr. Q. Zhu and colleagues at Shaoxing People's Hospital in China investigated the relationship between omega-3 PUFAs and insulin resistance in patients with type 2 diabetes and NAFLD. Their study involved 137 volunteers: fifty-one people with type 2 diabetes and NAFLD, fifty people with diabetes only, and forty-two healthy controls. The researchers found that blood levels of omega-3 PUFA are "negatively correlated with insulin resistance" and that a low level of "omega-3 PUFA plays a very important role in the development of diabetes mellitus" (Zhu, 2010).

MANAGING DIABETES

EPA/DHA supplements are not a cure for type 2 diabetes, but they are a healthy additive to an overall diabetes prevention and treatment plan. Drs. D. Fedor and D. Kelley of the University of California, Davis, summarize the role of EPA and DHA against prediabetes and diabetes: "Omega-3 PUFA supplementation has clinical significance in the prevention and reversal of insulin resistance. However, increased intake of omega-3 PUFAs should be part of an overall healthy lifestyle that includes weight control, exercise, and reduction in the intake of refined sugars, [and] omega-6, saturated, and trans fatty acids" (Fedor, 2009).

Studies have shown that an increased intake of EPA and DHA through diet and supplementation has positive effects on insulin activity, glucose control, blood lipids, obesity, and diabetes-related complications. Despite the fact that more definitive research has yet to be conducted on omega-3 LC-PUFAs and diabetes, we feel that diabetics and those with prediabetic conditions are among those who can benefit most from an intake of 1–2 grams of EPA and DHA every day!

Cancer

onventional chemotherapy drugs are often double-edged swords, as they kill the cancer cells but also damage the healthy cells, causing severe side effects and sometimes even death. EPA and DHA act as both a sword and a shield. In addition to being toxic to cancer cells, EPA and DHA protect healthy tissue by the favorable eicosanoids and docosanoids that they produce. Inflammation of tissue controlled by cytokines and other mediators provides a microenvironment for tumor growth and malignancy. Resolvins, protectins, and maresins made from EPA and DHA help counter that inflammation and may restrict cancerous cell growth. Scientific data indicate that EPA and DHA may inhibit the proliferation of cancer cells and work in synergy with chemotherapeutic drugs.

In this chapter we present studies showing that omega-3, long-chain polyunsaturated fatty acids (LC-PUFAs) may reduce the incidence of some cancers. We are not suggesting that they have a pronounced effect that directly prevents all types of cancer per se, but that they may have important indirect benefit for several types of cancer. Beside this, they may beneficially affect quality of life, better disease outcome, and physical activity in people with cancer.

THE DEVELOPMENT OF CANCER

Cancer is the uncontrolled growth of abnormal cells that can arise in any organ or tissue of the body. Whereas normal cells grow in an orderly, controlled pattern and at a predetermined rate, abnormal cells reproduce themselves endlessly even when new cells are not needed, causing a mass of abnormal cells (a tumor) to form. Tumors can be benign (noncancerous) or malignant (cancerous). Malignant tumors like the cells they are comprised of grow uncontrollably and spread (metastasize) by invading other tissues in the body. If the spread is not controlled, it can result in death.

There are more than 100 different types of cancer, affecting about 12 million Americans. The American Cancer Society (ACS) estimates that 1,638,910 new cancer cases will be diagnosed in 2012. This estimate does not include carcinoma in situ (noninvasive cancer) of any site except urinary bladder, and does not include basal and squamous cell skin cancers, which are not required to be reported to cancer registries. The ACS also

estimated that in 2012, about 577,190 Americans were expected to die of cancer, more than 1,500 people a day.

Cancer is the second most common cause of death in the United States, exceeded only by heart disease, accounting for nearly one of every four deaths. According to the ACS, cancer is caused by both external factors (tobacco, infectious organisms, chemicals, and radiation) and internal factors (inherited genetic mutations, hormones, immune conditions, and mutations to genes that occur from metabolism). These causal factors may act together or in sequence to initiate or promote the development of cancer. Ten or more years often pass between exposure to external factors and detectable cancer.

HOW EPA AND DHA MAY PROTECT AGAINST CANCER

The high-fish-consuming Inuits of Greenland not only have fewer incidences of heart disease, but their high omega-3 intake has also been found to lower their incidence of cancer. The same is true of high-fish-consuming Inuits in Alaska. In one study of the Alaskan Inuits, the occurrence of childhood cancer was found to be significantly lower compared to a North American population. Specifically, the incidence of neuroblastoma (a rare cancer of the sympathetic nervous system) was reduced tenfold from a million to 800,000 (only one-tenth of its former rate). In addition, Hodgkin's lymphoma, a cancer of the lymphatic system possibly related to infection and inflammation, was significantly reduced in this population (Lanier 2003).

Let's explore the possible mechanisms in EPA and DHA that may be at work here.

Inhibit Growth and Spread of Cancer Cells

Noting the change in incidence in breast cancer among Japanese women who Westernized their formerly high-fish diet, researchers began to suspect a relationship between decreased levels of EPA and DHA in the body and increased risk of breast cancer. In 1995 the body of science regarding omega-3 PUFAs and breast cancer was reviewed by researchers at the University of Kanazawa School of Medicine in Japan. They found that omega-3 PUFAs, primarily DHA and EPA, suppress the formation of breast cancer tumors and tumor cell proliferation, although the effect of DHA may be partly ascribed to increased amounts of EPA derived from DHA (Noguchi, 1995).

In 1997 Japanese researchers investigated DHA and EPA, including a series of omega-6 PUFAs for their anti-tumor and anti-metastatic effects. After implanting laboratory animals with rapidly growing colon cancer cells, the researchers observed that EPA and DHA significantly inhibited tumor growth at the implantation site and substantially decreased the numbers of nodules (lesions) that metastasized to the animals' lungs. Treatment with high doses of omega-6 linoleic acid (LA) increased the numbers of lung metastatic nodules. Interestingly, EPA and DHA only inhibited the lung colonizations when they were administered together with the tumor cells, suggesting that their protective effect is most influential when they are present in cells before tumor cells develop.

The researchers also found that tumor cells pretreated with fatty acids in vivo, in particular with DHA, helped to prevent the migration of cancer cells from spreading to the lung when transferred to new hosts. Thus, DHA treatment exerted marked antimetastatic activity associated with a pronounced change in the fatty acid component of tumor cells. The results indicate that uptake of DHA into tumor cells can alter tumor-cell membrane characteristics and decrease the cell's ability to metastasize (Iigo, 1997).

Human studies suggest that decreasing the ratio of omega-6 to omega-3 PUFAs decreases the risk of prostate cancer from developing and progressing. This was investigated in men undergoing radical prostatectomy who were randomly assigned to receive a low-fat diet with 5 grams of fish oil daily (a dietary omega-6/omega-3 ratio of 2:1) or a controlled Western diet (with an omega-6/omega-3 ratio of 15:1) for four to six weeks prior to surgery. After the surgery, men in the low-fat fish-oil group were found to have fewer tumors (both less benign and cancerous tissue) and slower cancer cell growth than men consuming the Westernized diet (Aronson, 2011).

Lower Breast Cancer Risk

A 2009 study at the South Korean National Cancer Center in Gyeonggi examined the association between fish and omega-3 intake with the risk of breast cancer in a case-controlled study of Korean women. This study included 358 women with breast cancer and 360 controls with no history of cancerous tumors. The women were given a food-frequency questionnaire to determine their dietary consumption of fish (fatty and lean fish) and intake of EPA and DHA. The study found that a high intake of fatty fish was associated with a reduced risk for breast cancer in both pre- and postmenopausal women (Kim, 2009).

Comparing women in the top 25 percent of EPA intake (101 milligrams [mg] or more daily) to those in the lowest 25 percent of EPA intake (14 mg or less daily) showed a 50 percent reduction in breast cancer risk. With DHA, women in the top 25 percent of DHA intake (213 mg or more daily) had only 44 percent of the breast cancer risk of those in the lowest 25 percent of DHA intake (37 mg or less daily).

The findings were different when looking at the risks specifically for premenopausal and postmenopausal women, but followed the same pattern with EPA and DHA lowering the risk of breast cancer. The risk of breast cancer for premenopausal women was reduced by 33 percent for those consuming the highest 25 percent of EPA intake (101 mg daily) compared to those in the lowest 25 percent of EPA intake (14 mg of less daily). For postmenopausal women, the risk of breast cancer was markedly reduced by 62 percent in the highest intake group (101 mg or more daily) compared to women in the lowest intake group (14 mg or less daily). The reasons for the differences in the protective effect of EPA between pre- and postmenopausal women are not clear, but the researchers offered several possible explanations. It is the results that count, more so than the mechanisms involved.

For DHA, the highest intake group (213 mg or more daily) had a 68 percent reduced risk of breast cancer for postmenopausal women. In other words, postmenopausal women had only 32 percent of the incidence of breast cancer than those in the lowest DHA group. Table 19.1 shows the decreased risk of developing breast cancer for each of the four intake ranges for EPA and DHA. The breast cancer reduction for all women in the study in the highest intake group was 56 percent compared to those in the lowest intake group.

TABLE 19.1. CONSUMPTION OF EPA AND DHA AND THE RISK OF BREAST CANCER		
DAILY INTAKE	REDUCED RISK OF BREAST CANCER	
EPA	ALL WOMEN	POSTMENOPAUSAL WOMEN
101 mg or more EPA	50%	62%
41–100 mg EPA	9%	22%
15–41 mg EPA	10%	19%
14 mg or less EPA	—	—
DHA		
213 mg or more DHA	56%	68%
92–212 mg DHA	23%	19%
38–91 mg DHA	14%	10%
37 mg or less DHA	—	—

Source: Based on data from Kim et al.

Based on these findings, the researchers concluded, "This investigation has identified fish and fish omega-3 fatty acid intake as an important potential protective factor in the nutritional etiology of breast cancer.

Our results revealed an inverse relation between breast cancer risk and dietary intake of fatty fish and omega-3 fatty acids from fish."

In 2004 Dr. M. Saadatian-Elahi and a team of researchers conducted a meta-analysis of studies that analyzed blood markers of fatty acids in association with breast cancer risk. Women with the greatest total omega-3 fatty acid, EPA, and DHA content in their blood had 39 percent, 31 percent, and 32 percent lower risk, respectively, of developing breast cancer. The analysis was based on three cohort and seven case-control studies involving 2,031 women and a control group of 2,334 women (Saadatian-Elahi, 2004).

Fish oil supplements have also demonstrated beneficial effects for protecting against breast cancer. In 2007 researchers from the Samuel Lunenfeld Research Institute at Mount Sinai Hospital in Toronto examined cod liver oil supplementation with breast cancer risk. They observed that consuming cod liver oil once a week or more during adolescence reduced the risk of developing breast cancer later in life by 24 percent. It is not clear whether vitamin D in the fish liver oil could explain some or all of the protective effect (Knight, 2007).

Inhibit Production of Inflammatory Compounds

In Chapter 4 we introduced a substance in cells called nuclear factor-κB (NF-κB), a master switch involved in the inflammatory process, and earlier in this chapter we mentioned the role of inflammation in cancer. The following study brings both of these concepts together. In 2010 Dr. E. White and her colleagues at the Fred Hutchinson Cancer Research Center in Seattle reported on findings from their six-year study of 35,016 postmenopausal women, which found that women who regularly took fish oil supplements were 32 percent less likely to develop ductal breast cancer, the most common type of the disease. The researchers noted, "Animal and human studies support fish oil as having anti-inflammatory and possibly other properties that could reduce breast cancer risk. Fish oil may be associated with a reduction of breast cancer risk because of its anti-inflammatory properties. EPA and DHA are thought to reduce inflammation by suppressing the production of NF-κB, including interleukin-6 (IL-6) and cyclooxygenase-2 (COX-2). Because EPA and DHA are incorporated into the phospholipids in the cell membrane at the expense of arachidonic acid (an omega-6 PUFA) when they are in balanced proportion to AA, EPA and DHA reduce the reservoir of arachidonic acid for COX-2 to synthesize pro-inflammatory prostaglandin E2. They concluded, "Fish oil may be inversely associated with breast cancer risk" (Brasky, 2010).

May Prevent Formation of Many Types of Cancers

Also in 2010, Drs. H. Gleissman, J. Johnsen, and P. Kogner of the Karolinska Institute in Sweden reviewed the growing body of scientific evidence and pronounced omega-3 PUFAs the "protectors of good and killers of evil." The scientists reviewed the results from numerous animal and human studies associating the consumption of omega-3 fatty acids with a decreased risk of cancers of the breast, prostate, colon, and kidneys (Smith-Warner, 2006; Wolk, 2006; Courtney, 2007; Fradet, 2009; Thiebaut, 2009). They also reviewed animal studies, specifically on DHA supplementation and cancer prevention, showing that DHA-enriched or fish oil-enriched diets can inhibit the formation of papillomas (benign growths) (Akihisa, 2004), and carcinogenesis of the mammary glands (Noguchi, 1997; Yuri, 2003; Manna, 2008) and of the large and small intestines, and lung (Toriyama-Baba, 2001). In addition to prevention of these cancers, DHA-enriched diets have also been shown to reduce the formation of aberrant crypt foci (one of the earliest changes in the lining of the colon and rectum that form before colorectal polyps) (Takahashi, 1993), colon cancer carcinoma (Iigo, 1997), sarcoma (a type of cancer that is rarer than carcinoma) (Ramos, 2004), and prostate cancer (Kelavkar, 2006).

In their discussion of the findings, the researchers pointed out that "dietary habits, and especially intake of fat, do more to the body than just influence waist circumference and weight. Dietary habits affect the system as a whole, down to gene level, and both the amount of fat and the kind of fat we eat can have significant effects on health. Actually, daily fat intake can be a matter of life and death on both a cellular and personal level." In concluding remarks, they asked, "May our current diet with [its] decreased omega-3/omega-6 ratio contribute to the increased cancer incidence, and could an omega-3-enriched diet be used as a preventive measure against cancer?" (Gleissman, 2010). Well, there is certainly good evidence to suggest that this is a distinct possibility.

Recent data suggest that omega-3 PUFAs may also play a role in cancer formation by counteracting the pro-cancer properties of soluble intercellular adhesion molecule-1 (sICAM-1). SICAM-1 is a specific type of cell adhesion molecule associated with both cancer formation and inflammation. This was investigated by including all first-incident cancer cases diagnosed in a large French study between 1994 and 2007. Researchers examined the impact of omega-3 PUFA intakes on sICAM-1 levels and cancer risk by comparing data from 408 people with cancer and 760 healthy controls. Their results linked higher omega-3 levels to lower sICAM-1 levels. This association was seen in people with four kinds of cancer, including breast and prostate cancer. In addition, higher blood levels of sICAM-1 were linked to higher cancer risk in people with below-average omega-3 intakes. Conversely, people with higher omega-3 intakes had lower sICAM-1 blood levels and lower risk of cancer, suggesting that omega-3 PUFA intake may counteract the pro-carcinogenic actions of sICAM (Touvier, 2012).

Thus, there is increasing support for an anti-cancer effect of EPA and DHA. Additionally, there are data showing that if cancer has developed, EPA/DHA supplementation may ease the way by decreasing inflammation, and as will be discussed shortly, decrease physical aspects of fatigue.

UNIQUE ROLE OF DHA IN CANCER PREVENTION AND TREATMENT

Epidemiological studies suggest that DHA is important in the prevention of several types of cancer, including cancers of the breast and brain (Larsson, 2004; Berquin, 2008).

Since DHA is so vital for brain and nerve cells, it has been looked at for help with brain cancer. DHA is the most abundant fatty acid in the brain and is vital to the health of nerve cell membranes. DHA, as discussed in Chapter 4, is metabolized by lipoxygenase enzymes, which through a series of steps eventually produce neuroprotectins and resolvins, potent anti-inflammatory and inflammation-resolving compounds. As such, DHA seems to be a good candidate to investigate for protection against brain cancer.

Targets Toxic Cancer Cells

Researchers at the Karolinska Institute in Sweden in conjunction with Harvard Medical School have found that DHA exerts anti-cancer effects and can induce cancer cell destruction in neuroblastoma, a childhood brain cancer that was mentioned at the start of this chapter (Gleissman, 2010). However, in neuroblastoma, the cancer protects itself from harm by shutting down the conversion of DHA into resolvins and neuroprotectins. One question then became, Could taking additional DHA overcome this protective action of the neuroblastoma?

Additional studies by Dr. H. Gleissman and colleagues examined a possible role of DHA in selectively killing cancer cells and not healthy cells. The researchers investigated whether supplementing animals with DHA affects the susceptibility of neuroblastoma cells (which are very resistant to chemotherapy) to oxidative stress in response to chemotherapy. DHA, but not the monounsaturated (omega-9) oleic acid, induced dose- and time-dependent neuroblastoma cell death. In other words, the more DHA and the longer it is taken, the more cancer cells die. The researchers concluded that their findings provide experimental evidence that DHA has the ability to kill neuroblastoma cancer cells that are resistant to chemotherapy drugs (Lindskog, 2006).

Increases Effectiveness and Eases Side Effects of Anti-Cancer Drugs

Surprisingly, DHA has been found to help those with cancer in another way. One small but impressive study examined the effect of DHA when combined with conventional drugs in breast cancer patients undergoing chemotherapy. The results indicated that incorporation of DHA can alter the treatment outcome.

In this study, twenty-five women with rapidly progressing breast cancer were supplemented with 1.8 grams of DHA daily during their chemotherapy treatments. The researchers measured the women's blood levels of

DHA and then divided them into high- and low-absorbing DHA groups. They then tracked the survival times of the women for approximately two and a half years. Women in the high-absorbing group survived 47 percent longer and had slower tumor progression compared to the women in the low-absorbing group (Bougnoux 2009).

Evidence suggests that inflammation may be a major contributing factor to the fatigue many cancer patients experience as a side effect of cancer and of standard treatment involving radiation and chemotherapy. Because research in healthy people has shown reduced inflammation with higher dietary intake of omega-3 PUFAs, investigators at the National Institutes of Health in Bethesda, Maryland, wanted to explore whether omega-3s could potentially reduce fatigue in breast cancer patients. The researchers recruited 633 breast cancer patients participating in the Health, Eating, Activity, and Lifestyle Study. The women completed a food-frequency/dietary-supplement questionnaire and provided a blood sample so C-reactive protein (CRP) and serum amyloid A protein (two markers of inflammation) could be measured thirty months after diagnosis. They also completed standard fatigue assessment tests (the Piper Fatigue Scale and Short Form-36 vitality scale) thirty-nine months after diagnosis. Women with high CRP levels were almost twice (1.8 times) as likely to experience fatigue. Women with higher intakes of omega-6 PUFAs relative to omega-3s had higher CRP levels and even greater odds of fatigue. Women with higher intakes of omega-3 PUFAs relative to omega-6s had less inflammation and less physical fatigue (Alfano, 2012).

Other side effects beside fatigue can occur during chemotherapy that can significantly impact one's quality of life. In a randomized clinical trial, a supplement containing 2 grams of EPA and 0.9 grams of DHA was found to improve quality of life and daily performance in forty lung cancer patients during multimodality treatment. The intervention group scored significantly higher on quality-of-life parameters, and on physical, cognitive, and social function than the control group after five weeks (van de Meij, 2011).

USING EPA AND DHA WITH CAUTIOUS OPTIMISM

Even though most but not all data point at a possible anti-cancer effect of EPA and DHA, caution should be expressed. For example, a recent meta-analysis of fish consumption and prostate cancer risk failed to demonstrate a protective effect of fish consumption against the development of prostate cancer, although there was a significant 63 percent reduction in risk of death from prostate cancer (Szymanski, 2010). One new study even found that high blood levels of omega-3 are associated with an increased risk for developing aggressive prostate cancer! The study, however, concludes that the findings are contrary to those expected from the pro- and anti-inflammatory effects of these fatty acids and suggest a greater complexity of effects of these nutrients with regard to prostate cancer risk (Brasky, 2011).

Since then, more data again point at a beneficial anti-cancer effect of omega-3s. In this case-controlled study comprised of 79 men with prostate cancer and 187 healthy controls, intakes of omega-6 and omega-3 fatty acids were determined using a food-frequency questionnaire. Caucasian men who had a high ratio of omega-6 to omega-3 fatty acids were at increased risk of developing prostate cancer, but not among African Americans. The risk was increased in all men, regardless of race, in those with rapidly progressing prostate cancer (Williams, 2011).

All in all, at this time, the evidence is building that 500–1,000 mg per day of EPA and DHA exert anti-proliferative effects on cancer cells and work in synergy with chemotherapeutic drugs. In the not-too-distant future, they may indeed become both a sword against cancer cells and a shield to protect healthy cells.

Guidelines and Dosages for Optimizing Your Health by Restoring EPA/DHA Levels

Our purpose in writing this book is that we hope your health can benefit from the nutritional treasure unlocked from the Eskimos. We have presented important facts about the benefits of EPA and DHA, which are so vital to health, but that have essentially disappeared or are dangerously dwindling from modern diets.

We began with Drs. Dyerberg's and Bang's adventures and discoveries in Arctic Greenland and continued through the latest research about several of the modern epidemics of diseases associated with the deficiency of omega-3, long-chain polyunsaturated fatty acids (LC-PUFAs). It is now widely recognized that EPA and DHA are protective against cardiovascular disease, stroke, macular degeneration, and arthritis. The importance of DHA and EPA to cognitive function and to mental health disorders such as depression and dementias including Alzheimer's disease is well established. The role of EPA and DHA in slowing the aging process and protecting against cancer is, like its effect on type 1 and 2 diabetes, under serious investigation.[3] What remains to be better understood by health advisors is that omega-3 LC-PUFAs are generally fundamental to health as well as to preventing disease.

JUST THE BEGINNING

This is just the beginning of the omega-3 story. We anticipate that as research continues, we will better understand the multiple roles of these essential nutrients. We anticipate greater understanding and expansion of our knowledge of how omega-3 LC-PUFAs can benefit people suffering from diseases beyond those discussed in this book. Already intriguing findings suggest that EPA and DHA can reduce the incidence of asthma and eczema in children when their mothers are better nourished with EPA and DHA during pregnancy. There is also limited support for the theory that the anti-inflammatory actions of EPA and DHA can lessen the severity of asthma in adults as well, but at this time, the studies are inconclusive. Clinical studies with better measurement of biomarkers will be required to make this determination.

Similarly, there is a likelihood it will be found that other diseases and disorders including attention deficit hyperactivity disorder (ADHD) and allergies may benefit from restoring EPA and DHA levels to optimal values. This is based on the knowledge that the health of every cell, every organ, and every system is affected by omega-3 LC-PUFAs.

As EPA and DHA are properly recognized as essential to health, dietary guidelines and recommendations will reflect their need. In the United States, at this writing, EPA and DHA are not recognized as being dietary essential, although they are in several other countries. Those countries have issued official dietary recommendations for EPA plus DHA that range from 200 to 500 milligrams (mg) per day. In 2002 the Institute of Medicine, a part of the Academy of Sciences, concluded that insufficient data were available to define Dietary Reference Intakes (DRIs) for EPA or DHA.

As research began growing almost exponentially, in 2008, the Technical Committee on Dietary Lipids of the International Life Sciences Institute of North America sponsored a workshop to examine whether the evidence specific to the major chronic diseases in the United States —coronary heart disease, cancer, and cognitive decline—had evolved sufficiently to

---

3. In the previous chapters on the clinical uses of EPA and DHA, researchers studied various forms of omega-3 fatty acids. Sometimes they investigated the actions of only specific PUFAs, such as EPA or DHA or both. At other times, they investigated larger groups of PUFAs, such as all omega-3 PUFAs (not just EPA and/or DHA), and occasionally they studied all PUFAs, including all omega-3s and omega-6s. What is important to bear in mind is that no matter which form of omega-3 was studied, EPA and DHA are the most important and most bioactive of the omega-3 fatty acids.

justify establishing a DRI for EPA and DHA. Based on the workshop's determinations, the Institute concluded:

1. Consistent evidence from multiple research paradigms demonstrates a clear, inverse relation between EPA plus DHA intake and risk of fatal (and possibly nonfatal) CHD [coronary heart disease] that supports a DRI for EPA plus DHA between 250 and 500 mg per day.

2. Because of the low conversion from dietary ALA, protective tissue levels of EPA plus DHA can be achieved only through direct consumption of these fatty acids.

3. Evidence of EPA plus DHA's beneficial effects on cognitive decline are emerging but are not yet sufficient to support recommendation of an intake level different from that needed to achieve CHD risk reduction.

4. EPA plus DHA do not appear to reduce cancer risk. [We present information in support of a beneficial relationship in Chapter 19.]

5. There is no evidence that intakes of EPA plus DHA in these recommended ranges are harmful (Harris, 2009).

The parent omega-3 alpha-linolenic acid (ALA) is recognized as being dietary essential, but that is mostly because some ALA can be converted into EPA and DHA. There is, at this writing, no other known critical function of ALA other than its conversion to EPA and DHA. The limited conversion of ALA to EPA allows life to exist, but not at its optimal level. This can be achieved only with optimal dietary intake of EPA and DHA. As nutritionists recognize that it is the omega-3 LC-PUFAs themselves (EPA and DHA), and not other fatty acids, that have their own essential actions, including cellular membrane function and the formation of messenger and signaling molecules such as eicosanoids and docosanoids, the Western diet can be shifted back toward that of our ancestors, which works better with our genes. In the future, EPA and DHA will take their place alongside essential vitamins and minerals.

FREQUENTLY ASKED QUESTIONS

Why take fish oil and not eat more fish?

We advise consuming ample fatty fish in the diet, prepared without frying, as well as EPA and DHA supplements, when eating less than two to three (fatty) fish meals per week. Natural foods are always the best source of nutrients as they contain many nutrients and accessory factors. However, it is difficult for many people to obtain adequate amounts of EPA and DHA solely through their diet. Supplements help assure a known quantity of EPA and DHA and can be consumed conveniently on a daily basis. Not all fish are rich in EPA and DHA. As we have mentioned elsewhere, good fish sources of EPA and DHA are the cold-water fatty fish including mackerel, salmon, herring, tuna, and sardines that live naturally in open waters rich in the natural sources of EPA and DHA in phytoplankton.

Are all forms of fish preparation equal?

No! Fried fish are unwanted. Broiled or baked fish are protective. As we pointed out in the inset on page 119, not only are fried fish not protective, but they seem to be a contributing factor to stroke as well.

How much EPA and DHA should I take?

This depends on your objective and the quality of your diet. The American Heart Association recommends eating fish (particularly fatty fish) at least two times (two servings) a week. Each serving is 3.5 ounces cooked, or about three-fourths cup of flaked fish. Fatty fish like salmon, mackerel, herring, lake trout, sardines, and albacore tuna are high in omega-3 fatty acids. Increasing omega-3 fatty acid consumption through foods is preferable. However, those with coronary artery disease—and those with health problems other than heart diseases—may not get enough omega-3 by diet alone. These people may want to take supplements.

Generally, if you are in good health and are eating a healthful diet, consider taking about 500 mg of EPA/DHA combined daily either from your food alone or from supplements. This is not the same as saying, "Take 500 mg of fish oil." Fish oils vary in their concentration of EPA and DHA. They contain other good nutrients in addition to EPA and DHA such as vitamins, other omega-3 PUFAs, and monounsaturated fatty acids. Read the label closely and determine how much EPA and DHA are present in each serving. To best maintain good health, the total intake of EPA and DHA should be about 500–1,000 mg.

For specific conditions, the following are useful guidelines based on the 2012 body of science. Future research may change these recommendations. Also, the advice of your personal health practitioner should be followed if it is not in accordance with these general guidelines:

CONDITION	SUGGESTED DAILY DOSAGE OF EPA/DHA IN MILLIGRAMS (mg)
Aging (for prevention)	500–1,000 mg
Alzheimer's and dementia	1,000–2,000 mg
Arthritis (for pain relief)	3,000 mg
Bipolar disorder and schizophrenia	2,000–3,000 mg
Cancer	500–1,000 mg*
Diabetes and prediabetes	1,000–2,000 mg
Heart attacks	1,000 mg
High triglycerides	2,000–4,000 mg
Memory and cognition (for maintenance)	500 mg
Mood disorder	500–2,000 mg
Pregnancy (for healthy fetal development) and first three months after birth	200–300 mg (of DHA)
Stroke	500 mg*
Vision problems (for macular degeneration and dry eye syndrome)	500–1,000 mg

*Note: The recommended intakes are safe and most probably beneficial, but future science may adjust our knowledge. If supplementing with EPA/DHA to help with more than one condition, take the higher of the dosages listed.

Should I take my EPA and DHA as fish oil, krill oil, or calamarine oil, or from algae and related microorganisms?

It doesn't matter. This book describes the research behind the omega-3 LC-PUFAs EPA and DHA. The results reported are for EPA and DHA, which are the same no matter what their source. Be sure to read the labels to make sure you are getting appropriate amounts of EPA plus DHA.

Is it better to take the triglyceride form or purified ester form of EPA and DHA?

Most fatty acids in the body, as well as in fish, vegetables, fruits, and other animals, are found in the triglyceride form. The vast majority of fish oil products are in the natural triglyceride form. It really makes little difference. Studies have shown that even if the triglyceride form is absorbed somewhat better than the ethyl ester form, both forms are well absorbed and function in your body (Dyerberg, 2010). What is important is the total amount of EPA and DHA.

What is the difference between fish body oil and fish liver oil?

Commercial sources of EPA include fish body oil. This is extracted from the whole body of fatty, cold-water fish that is especially rich in EPA and DHA. This fish oil should not be confused with fish liver oils such as cod liver oil. Cod liver oil is an excellent dietary supplement that has been used for many generations to promote the health of children and even in adults to help against arthritis. Modern cod liver oils are rich sources of EPA and DHA as a teaspoon contains about 400 mg of EPA and 500 mg of DHA. The health benefits described in this book pertain to EPA and DHA at the level of about 1 gram and more. Cod liver oil also contains large amounts of fat-soluble vitamins A and D. One teaspoon of cod liver oil contains about 850 international units (IU) of vitamin A, which is 17 percent of the 8,000 IU DRI for this vitamin, and about 400 IU of vitamin D. The upper limit of dietary intake without any reported adverse effect is currently 2,000 IU per day for vitamin D by the Institute of Medicine (although many consider it non-toxic at 10,000 IU per day). Therefore, supplementation of these vitamins in conjunction with cod liver oil (in the dosages we recommend) is not suggested.

Are flaxseeds, flaxseed oil, and other seeds and oils good sources of EPA and DHA?

We have stressed that all omega-3 PUFAs are good for you, but they are all not equal. Only EPA and DHA can be formed into the eicosanoids and docosanoids and related compounds that have many effects in the body. As we have discussed in earlier chapters, short- and medium-chain fatty acids can only be converted into EPA and DHA on a very limited basis that is inadequate for optimal health. As stated in the *American Journal of Clinical Nutrition,* "Given the typical Western diet, even large doses of ALA—found in flaxseeds, flaxseed oil, and other seeds and oils—result in only small increases in plasma EPA, and no effect on DHA" (Arterburn, 2006). However, ingestion of vegetable oils such as those enriched in the eighteen-carbon chain, four-double bond stearidonic acid (SDA) increases EPA concentration but not DHA levels.

Should I take DHA for mental health and EPA for heart health?

You need to protect both your cardiovascular system and your brain and nervous system. Therefore, you should take both so that together they reach the appropriate levels. For general health, this means you should take at least 500–1,000 mg of EPA and DHA. People consuming supplements that are either EPA only or DHA only should be sure to consume complementary EPA or DHA from other sources. In the total of 1,000 mg of EPA and DHA a day, there should be a minimum of 200–300 mg per day of each in the total diet.

When should I take fish oil?

Fish oil is best taken with meals.

What about burping or belching?

Some people, such as those who have had their gall bladders removed, can be bothered by belching or burping after consuming any oil. If someone finds this a problem, you can often prevent it by dividing dosages into two or three a day instead of all at once. Be sure to keep the fish oil fresh after opening by storing it in the refrigerator.

What if I am allergic to seafood?

Allergies can result from the proteins in foods. Oils do not contain proteins. However, if you are allergic to seafood, proceed cautiously or use a source derived from algae or related microorganisms.

Will I smell fishy if I take fish oil?

Not with today's purified fish oils.

Is fish oil contaminated with mercury, lead, and other harmful toxins?

Harmful environmental toxins like methylmercury, lead, polychlorinated biphenyls (PCBs), and dioxins can concentrate in fish flesh, but fish oil is purified to remove toxins. Fish oil sold by major, long-standing manufacturers is processed to the high standards of the omega-3 trade group, the Global Organization of EPA and DHA (GOED).

Are there any adverse effects I may experience from taking EPA and DHA?

The Norwegian Scientific Committee for Food Safety (VKM) studied dosage levels and effects of fish oil for adverse effects including bleeding times, lipid peroxidation, inflammation and immunity, and glucose metabolism and gastrointestinal disturbances. They found that adverse effects were not present below 6,900 mg (6.9 grams) for bleeding times. The report concluded, "Negative health effects regarding gastrointestinal function, including abdominal cramps, flatulence, eructation, vomiting and diarrhea, have been reported, but seem to be associated with intake of an oily substance and not ascribed specifically to EPA and/or DHA. Based on the reviewed literature, it is not possible to identify clear adverse effects from EPA and/or DHA, which can be used for setting tolerable upper intake levels" (VKM, 2011). GOED notes that normal intakes of EPA and DHA (such as we recommend in this book) are safe, and even at the higher pharmaceutical dosages in use today, only minor issues have been observed.

IN CLOSING

It's been a long journey from the Arctic to the many laboratories and clinics around the world that today are helping to develop the omega-3 story, which is our inheritance of the nutritional treasure of the Greenland Eskimos. Hopefully, understanding the uniqueness and essentialness of EPA and DHA will help improve the health of millions of people. As we conclude this book, Dr. Dyerberg reflected and remarked, "It has been a privilege and a blessing to have had the good fortune to introduce into human nutrition a new and healthy nutrient." To which I added, "You have brought to us the greatest nutritional discovery since the discovery of vitamins nearly a century ago."

Be well and live better longer!

References

Chapter 1

Bang HO, et al. Plasma lipid and lipoprotein pattern in Greenlandic West-Coast Eskimos, *Lancet* 1971;1(7710):1143–1145.

Dyerberg J, et al. Fatty acid composition of plasma lipids in Greenland Eskimos. *AJCN* 1975;28:958–966.

Chapter 2

Burr GO, Burr MM. A new deficiency disease produced by the rigid exclusion of fat from the diet. *Biol Chem* 1929;82:345–367.

Burr GO, Burr MM. The nature and role of the fatty acids essential in nutrition. *Biol Chem* 1930;86:587–621.

Enig M. *Know Your Fats*. Silver Spring, MD: Bethesda Press, 2000, 17, 112.

Plourde M, Cunnane SC. Extremely limited synthesis of long-chain polyunsaturates in adults: implications for their dietary essentiality and use as supplements. *Appl Physiol Nutr Metab* 2007;32:619–634.

Stillwell W, Wassall SR. Docosahexaenoic acid: membrane properties of a unique fatty acid. *Chem Phys Lipids* 2003;126:1–27.

Chapter 3

Danaei GM, et al. The preventable causes of death in the united sates: comparative risk assessment of dietary, lifestyle, and metabolic risk factors. *PLoS Med* 2009; 6(4): e1000058. Epub 2009 Apr 28.

Chapter 4

Lee TH, Menica-Huerta JM, Shih C, et al. Characterization and biologic properties of 5,12-dihydroxy derivatives of eicosapentaenoic acid, including leukotriene B5 and the double lipoxygenase product. *J Biol Chem* 1984;259(4):2383–2389.

Magee P, Pearson S, Whittingham-Dowd J, et al. PPAR? as a molecular target of EPA anti-inflammatory activity during TNF-α-impaired skeletal muscle cell differentiation. *J Nutr Biochem* 2012 Feb 1. [Epub ahead of print]

Micallef MA, Munro IA, Garg ML, et al. An inverse relationship between plasma n-3 fatty acids and C-reactive protein in healthy individuals. *Eur J Clin Nutr* 2009;63:1154–1156.

Phang M, Lincz L, Seldon M, et al. Acute supplementation with eicosapentaenoic acid reduces platelet microparticle activity in healthy subjects. *J Nutr Biochem* 2011 Nov 30. [Epub ahead of print]

Reinders I, Virtanen JK, Brouwer IA, et al. Association of serum n-3 polyunsaturated fatty acids with C-reactive protein in men. *Eur J Clin Nutr* 2011 Nov 23. [Epub ahead of print]

Serhan CN, Hong S, Grornert K, et al. Resolvins: a family of bioactive products of omega-3 fatty acid transformation circuits initiated by aspirin treatment that counter proinflammation signals. *J Exp Med* 2002;196:1025–1037.

Serhan CN, Petasis NA. Resolvins and protectins in inflammation resolution. *Chem Rev* 2011;111(10):5922–5943.

Serhan CN. Novel lipid mediators and resolution mechanisms in acute inflammation: to resolve or not? *Am J Pathol* 2010 Oct;177(4):1576–1591.

Chapter 5

Arterburn LM, Hall EB, Oken H. Distribution, interconversion, and dose response of n-3 fatty acids in humans. *Am J Clin Nutr* 2006;83(6 Suppl):1467S–1476S.

Bowman GL, Silbert LC, Howieson D, et al. Nutrient biomarker patterns, cognitive function, and MRI measures of brain aging. *Neurology* 2012 Jan 24;78:241–249.

Brenna TJ, Salem N, Sinclair AJ, et al. α-linolenic acid supplementation and conversion to n-3 long-chain polyunsaturated fatty acids in humans. ISSFAL. Official statatement number 5, March 2009. Available online at: http://archive.issfal.org/index.php/lipid-matters-mainmenu-8/issfal-policy-statements-mainmenu-9/164-aladha-bioequivalence.

National Cholesterol Education Program (NCEP) Expert Panel. Total PUFA account for about 7% of total calories in the average American diet. Third Report of the NCEP Expert Panel on Detection, Evaluation, and Treatment of High Blood Cholesterol in Adults (Adult Treatment Panel III) final report. *Circulation* 2002 Dec 17;106(25): 3143–3421.

Whelan J. Dietary stearidonic acid is a long chain (n-3) polyunsaturated fatty acid with potential health benefits. *J Nutr* 2009 Jan;139(1):5–10.

Wright JD, Wang CY, Kennedy-Stephenson J, et al. Dietary intake of ten key nutrients for public health, United States 1999–2000. Advance data from Vital Health Statistics; no. 334. Hyattsville: National Center for Health Statistics, 2003.

Chapter 6

Agricultural Research Service, United States Department of Agriculture. What we eat in America, NHANES 2007–2008 (rev. 2010). Available online at: www.ars.usda.gov/sp2userfiles/place/12355000/pdf/0708/table_1_nin_gen_07.pdf.

Blasbalg TL, Hibbeln JR, Ramsden CE, et al., Changes in consumption of omega-3 and omega-6 fatty acids in the United States during the 20th century. *Am J Clin Nutr* 2011 May;93(5):950–962.

Conference on Health Effects of Polyunsaturated Fatty Acids in Seafoods (1985: Washington, D.C.) . Health effects of polyunsaturated fatty acids in seafoods. AP Simopoulos, RR Kifer, RE Martin, eds. Imprint Orlando: Academic Press, 1986.

Dolecek TA, Grandits G. Health effects of w3 polyunsaturated fatty acids in seafood. *World Rev Nutr Diet* 1991;66:205–216.

Harris WS, Mozaffarian D, Lefevre M, et al. Towards establishing dietary reference intakes for eicosapentaenoic and docosahexaenoic acids. *J Nutr* 2009 Apr;139(4): 804S–819S.

Chapter 7

Bang HO, Dyerberg J, Nielsen AB. Plasma lipid and lipoprotein pattern in Greenlandic West Coast Esikos. *Lancet* Apr 1971;1(7701):1143–1146.

De Caterina, R. n–3 fatty acids in cardiovascular disease. *N Engl J Med* 2011; 364:2439–2450.

Chapter 8

Albert CM, Campos H, Stampfer M, et al. Blood levels of long-chain n-3 fatty acids and the risk of sudden death. *N Engl J Med* 2002 Apr 11; 346:1113–1118.

American Heart Association Science. Advisory and Coordinating Committee on May 28, 2002 and published in great detail in the journal *Circulation* 2002;106:2747.

Bansal S, Buring JE, Rifai N, et al. Fasting compared with nonfasting triglycerides and risk of cardiovascular events in women. *JAMA* 2007;298(3):309–316.

Belin RJ, Greenland P, Martin L, et al. Fish intake and the risk of incident heart failure: the Women's Health Initiative. *Circ Heart Fail* 2011 May 24. [Epub ahead of print]

Bernstein AM, Ding EL, Willett WC, et al. A meta-analysis shows that docosahexaenoic acid from algal oil reduces serum triglycerides and increases HDL-cholesterol and LDL-cholesterol in persons without coronary heart disease. *J Nutr* 2012 Jan;142(1):99-104.

Bhalodkar NC, Blum S, Rana T, et al. Comparison of high-density and low-density lipoprotein cholesterol subclasses and sizes in Asian-Indian women with caucasian women. *Clin Cardiol* 2005;28:247–251.

Burr ML, et al. Diet and Reinfarction Trial (DART): design, recruitment, and compliance. *Eur Heart J* 1989;10(6):558–567.

Burr ML, et al. Effects of changes in fat, fish, and fibre intakes on death and myocardial reinfarction: Diet and Reinfarction Trial (DART). *Lancet* 1989;2(8666):757–761.

Danaei G, Ding EL, Mozaffarian D, et al. The preventable causes of death in the United States: comparative risk assessment of dietary, lifestyle, and metabolic risk factors. *PLoS Med* 2009;6(4):e1000058.

de Goede J, Geleijnse JM, et al. Marine (n-3) fatty acids, fish consumption, and the 10-year risk of fatal and nonfatal coronary heart disease in a large population of dutch adults with low fish intake. *J Nutr* 2010;140(5):1023–1028.

Dolecek TA, Grandits G. Health effects of w3 polyunsaturated fatty acids in seafood. *World Rev Nutr Diet* 1991;66:205–216.

Einvik G, Klemsdal TO, Sandvick L, et al. A randomized clinical trial on n-3 polyunsaturated fatty acids supplementation and all-cause mortality in elderly men at high cardiovascuclar risk. *Eur J Cardiovasc Prev Rehabil* 2010 Oct;17(5):588–592.

Farzaneh-Far R, et al. Association of marine omega-3 fatty acid levels with telomeric aging in patients with coronary heart disease. *JAMA* 2010;303(3):250–257.

Farzaneh-Far R. et al. Telomere length trajectory and its determinants in persons with coronary artery disease: longitudinal findings from the Heart and Soul Study. *PLoS One* 2010;5(1): e8612.

Fritsch D, et al. A multicenter study of the effect of dietary supplementation with fish oil omega-3 fatty acids on carprofen dosage in dogs with osteoarthritis. *J Amer Veterinary Medical Assoc* 2010;236(5):535–539.?

Galarraga B, et al. Cod liver oil (n-3 fatty acids) as a non-steroidal anti-inflammatory drug sparing agent in rheumatoid arthritis. *Rheumatol* 2008;47:665–669.?

GISSI-Prevenzione Investigators. Dietary supplementation with n-3 polyunsaturated fatty acids and vitamin e after myocardial infarction: results of the GISSI-Prevenzione Trial. *Lancet* 1999;354:447–455.

Harris, WS. Extending the cardiovascular benefits of omega-3 fatty acids. *Curr Atheroscler Rep* 2005 Sep;7(5):375-380; 2009 update available online at www.joslinresearch.org/eventnet/pdfSeminar/LibbyPaper2.pdf.

Harris, WS. The omega-3 index: as a risk factor for coronary heart disease. *Am J Clin Nutr* 2008;87(6):1997S–2002S.

Harris WS. The omega-3 index: from biomarker to risk marker to risk factor. *Curr Atheroscler Rep* 2009 Nov;11(6):411–417.

Harris WS, Kris-Etherton PM, Harris KA. Intakes of long-chain omega-3 fatty acid associated with reduced risk for death from coronary heart disease in healthy adults. *Curr Atheroscler Rep* 2008 Dec;10(6):503–509.

Harris WS, Mozaffarian D, Lefevre M, et al. Towards establishing dietary reference intakes for eicosapentaenoic and docosahexaenoic acids. *J Nutr* 2009 Apr;139(4): 804S–819S.

Harris WS, von Schacky C. The omega-3 index: a new risk factor for death from CHD. *Prev Med* 2004;39:212–220.

Heidt MC, Vician M, Stracke SK, et al. Beneficial effects of intravenously administered n-3 fatty acids for the prevention of atrial fibrillation after coronary artery bypass surgery: a prospective randomized study. *Thorac Cardiovasc Surg* 2009 Aug;57:5: 276–280.

Hubbard, WK. Letter responding to health claim petition dated November 3, 2003 (Martek Petition): omega-3 fatty acids and reduced risk of coronary heart disease (Docket No. 2003Q–0401). FDA Food. Available online at: www.fda.gov/Food/LabelingNutrition/LabelClaims/QualifiedHealthClaims/ucm072932.htm; see also, FDA announces qualified health claims for omega-3 fatty acids. Press Release P04-89 September 8, 2004. Available online at: www.fda.gov/SiteIndex/ucm108351.htm

Itomura M, Fujioka S, Hamazaki K, et al. Factors influencing EPA and DHA levels in red blood cells in Japan. *In Vivo* 2008;22:131–136.

Keaney JF. Immune modulation of atherosclerosis. *Circulation* 2011;124:559–560.

Kromhout D, Giltay EJ, Geleijnse JM. N-3 Fatty acids and cardiovascular events after myocardial infarction. *N Engl J Med* 2010; 363:2015–2027.

Kumar S, Sutherland F, et al. Effects of chronic omega-3 polyunsaturated fatty acid supplementation on human atrial mechanical function after reversion of atrial arrhythmias to sinus rhythm: reversal of tachycardia mediated atrial cardiomyopathy with fish oils. *Heart Rhythm* 2011 May;8(5):643–649.

Kumar S, Sutherland F, Morton JB, et al. Long term omega-3 polyunsaturated fatty acid supplementation reduces the recurrence of persistent atrial fibrillation after electrical cardioversion. *Heart Rhythm* 2012 Apr;9(4):483-491.

Kumar S, Sutherland F, Rosso R, et al. Effects of chronic omega-3 polyunsaturated fatty acid supplementation on human atrial electrophysiology. *Heart Rhythm* 2011 Apr;8(4):562–568.

Leaf A, Albert CM, Josephson M, et al. Prevention of fatal arrhythmias in high-risk subjects by fish oil n-3 fatty acid intake. *Circulation* 2005;112:2762–2768.

Lee SH, Shin MJ, Kim JS, et al. Blood eicosapentaenoic acid and docosahexaenoic acid as predictors of all-cause mortality in patients with acute myocardial infarction—data from Infarction Prognosis Study (IPS) Registry. *Circ J* 2009 Dec;73(12):2250–2257.

Leon H, Shibata MC, Sivakumaran S, et al. Effect of fish oil on arrhythmias and mortality: systematic review. *BMJ* 2008;337:a2931.

Libby P, Ridker PM, Maseri, A. Inflammation and atherosclerosis. *Circulation* 2002; 105:1135–43.

Macchia A, Monte S, Pelligrini F, et al. Omega-3 fatty acid supplementation reduces one-year risk of atrial fibrillation in patients hospitalized with myocardial infarction. *Eur J Clin Pharmacol* 2008 Jun;64(6):627–634.

Musa-Veloso K, Binns MA, Kocenas A, et al. Impact of low v. moderate intakes of long-chain n-3 fatty acids on risk of coronary heart disease. *Br J Nutr* 2011 Oct;106(8): 1129–1141.

National Institute for Health and Clinical Excellence (NICE). Secondary prevention in primary and secondary care for patients following a myocardial infarction. NICE clinical guideline 48, May 2007. Avaiable online at: www.nice.org.uk/nicemedia/pdf/CG48 NICEGuidance.pdf.

NHANES III Series 11 No. 2A. Electrocardiogram, dietary recall, laboratory, dietary supplement and prescription drug. National Center for Health Statistics, 1998. Available online at www.cdc.gov/nchs/about/major/nhanes/nh3data.htm.

NHANES III Series 11, No 3A, July 1999. Second exam files for dietary recall, examination, laboratory, additional laboratory analyses. National Center for Health Statistics, 1999. Available online at www.cdc.gov/nchs/about/major/nhanes/nh3data.htm.

Nordestgaard BG, Benn M, Schnohr P, et al. Nonfasting triglycerides and risk of myocardial infarction, ischemic heart disease, and death in men and women. *JAMA* 2007; 298(3):299–308.

Pase MP, Grima NA, et al. Do long-chain n-3 fatty acids reduce arterial stiffness? A meta-analysis of randomized controlled trials. *Br J Nutr* 2011 Oct 14;106:974–980.

Phang M, Lincz L, Seldon M, et al. Acute supplementation with eicosapentaenoic acid reduces platelet microparticle activity in healthy subjects. *J Nutr Biochem* 2011 Nov 30. [Epub ahead of print]

Schaefer EJ, Bongard V, Beiser AS, et al. Plasma phosphatidylcholine docosahexaenoic acid content and risk of dementia and Alzheimer disease: the Framingham Heart Study. *Arch Neurol* 2006;63(11):1545–1550.

Siscovick DS, Raghunathan TE, King I, et al. Dietary intake and cell membrane levels of long-chain n-3 polyunsaturated fatty acids and the risk of primary cardiac arrest. *J Am Med Assoc.* 1995;274:1363–1367.

Skulas-Ray AC, Kris-Etherton PM, Harris WS, et al. Dose-response effects of omega-3 fatty acids on triglycerides, inflammation, and endothelial function in healthy persons with moderate hypertriglyceridemia. *Am J Clin Nutr* 2011;93(2):243–252.

Stensvold I, Tverdal A, Urdal P, et al. Non-fasting serum triglyceride concentration and mortality from coronary heart disease and any cause in middle aged Norwegian women. *BMJ* 1993;307:1318–1322.

Strøm M, Halldorsson TI, Mortensen EL, et al. Fish, n-3 fatty acids, and cardiovascular diseases in women of reproductive age: a prospective study in a large national cohort. *Hypertension* 2012 Jan;59(1):36–43.

Studer M, Briel M, Leimenstoll B, et al. Effect of different antilipidemic agents and diets on mortality: a systematic review. *Arch Intern Med* 2005;165: 725–730.

Tull SP, Yates CM, Maskrey BH, et al. Omega-3 fatty acids and inflammation: novel interactions reveal a new step in neutrophil recruitment. *PLoS Biology* 2009 Aug 25;7(8): e1000177.

Vedtofte MS, Jakobsen MU, Lauritzen L, et al. Dietary ?-linolenic acid, linoleic acid, and n-3 long-chain PUFA and risk of ischemic heart disease. *Am J Clin Nutr* 2011 Oct;94(4):1097–1103.

Virtanen JK, Mursu J, Voutilainen S, et al. Serum long-chain n-3 polyunsaturated fatty acids and risk of hospital diagnosis of atrial fibrillation in men. *Circulation* 2009 Dec 8;120(23):2315–2321.

Wang C, Chung M, Lichtenstein A, et al. *Effects of omega-3 fatty acids on cardiovascu-*

lar disease. Evidence Report/Technology Assessment No 94. AHRQ Pub No 04-E009-1. Rockville, MD: Agency for Healthcare Research and Quality, 2004.

Weber A and PC. Cardiovascular effects of omega 3 fatty acids. *NJM* 1988;318:549–557.

Wu JH, Lemaitre RN, King IB, et al. Association of plasma phospholipid long-chain omega-3 fatty acids with incident atrial fibrillation in older adults: the Cardiovascular Health Study. *Circulation* 2012 Mar 6;125(9)1084–1093.

Zhao YT, Chen Q, Sun YX, et al. Prevention of sudden cardiac death with omega-3 fatty acids in patients with coronary heart disease: a meta-analysis of randomized controlled trials. *Ann Med* 2009;41(4):301–310.

Chapter 9

Belayev L, Khoutorova L, Atkins KD, et al. Docosahexaenoic acid therapy of experimental ischemic stroke *Transl Stroke Res* 2011 Mar;2(1):33-41.

Freiberg JJ, Tybjaerg-Hansen A, Jensen JS, et al. Nonfasting triglycerides and risk of ischemic stroke in the general population. *JAMA* 2008;300(18):2142–2152.

He K, Rimm EB, Merchant A, et al. Fish consumption and risk of stroke in men. *JAMA* 2002 Dec 25;288(24):3130–3136.

He K, Song Y, Daviglus ML, et al. Fish consumption and incidence of stroke: a meta-analysis of cohort studies. *Stroke* 2004 Jul;35(7):1538–1542.

Hino A, Adachi H, Toyomasu K, et al. Very long-chain N-3 fatty acids intake and carotid atherosclerosis: an epidemiological study evaluated by ultrasonography. *Atherosclerosis* 2004 Sep;176(1):145–149.

Iso H, Rexrode KM, Stampfer MJ, et al. Intake of fish and omega-3 fatty acids and risk of stroke in women. *JAMA* 2001;285(3):304–312.

Jicha GA, Markesbery WR. Omega-3 fatty acids: potential role in the management of early Alzheimer's disease. *Clin Interv Aging* 2010 Apr 7;5:45–61.

Kashiyama T, Ueda Y, Nemoto T, et al. Relationship between coronary plaque vulnerability and serum n-3/n-6 polyunsaturated fatty acid ratio. *Circ J* 2011 Sep 22;75(10): 2432–2438.

Lalancette-Hebert M, Julien C, Cordeau P, et al. Accumulation of dietary docosahexaenoic acid in the brain attenuates acute immune response and development of postischemic neuronal damage. Stroke 2011 Aug 18. [Epub ahead of print]

Larsson SC, Orsini, N. Fish consumption and the risk of stroke: a dose-response meta-analysis. *Stroke* 2011 Dec;42(12):3621–3623.

Mozaffarian D, Longstreth WT, Lemaitre RN, et al. Fish consumption and stroke risk in elderly individuals: the cardiovascular health study. *Arch Intern Med* 2005 Jan 24;165(2):200–2006.

Nahab F, Le A, Judd S, et al. Racial and geographic differences in fish consumption: the REGARDS study. *Neurology* 2011 Jan 11;76(2):154–158.

Park Y, Park S, Yi H., et al. Low level of n-3 polyunsaturated fatty acids in erythrocytes is a risk factor for both acute ischemic and hemorrhagic stroke in Koreans. *Nutr Res* 2009 Dec;29(12):825–830.

Skulas-Ray AC, Kris-Etherton PM, Harris WS, et al. Dose-response effects of omega-3 fatty acids on triglycerides, inflammation, and endothelial function in healthy persons with moderate hypertriglyceridemia. *Am J Clin Nutr* 2011;93(2):243–252.

Tanaka K, Ishikawa Y, Yokoyama M, et al. Reduction in the recurrence of stroke by eicosapentaenoic acid for hypercholesterolemic patients: sub-analysis of the JELIS trial. *Stroke* 2008 Jul;39(7):2052–2058.

Thies F, Garry JM, Yaqoob P, et al. Association of n-3 polyunsaturated fatty acids with stability of atherosclerotic plaques: a randomised controlled trial. *Lancet* 2003 Feb 8;361(9356):477–485.

Chapter 10

Assies J, Lieverse R, Vreken P, et al. Significantly reduced docosahexaenoic and docosapentaenoic acid concentrations in erythrocyte membranes from schizophrenic patients compared with a carefully matched control group. *Biol Psychiatry* 2001; 49: 510–522.

Brantsæter AL, Birgisdottir BE, Meltzer HM, et al. Maternal seafood consumption and infant birth weight, length and head circumference in the Norwegian Mother and Child Cohort Study. *Br J Nutr* 2012 Feb;107(3):436–444.

Donahue SM, Rifas-Shiman SL, Gold DR, et al. Prenatal fatty acid status and child adiposity at age 3 y: results from a US pregnancy cohort. *Am J Clin Nutr* 2011 Apr;93(4): 780–788.

European Food Safety Authority Panel on Dietetic Products, Nutrition, and Allergies. Scientific opinion on dietary reference values for fats, including saturated fatty acids, polyunsaturated fatty acids, monounsaturated fatty acids, trans fatty acids, and cholesterol. *EFSA Journal* 2010;8(3):1461.

Hibbeln JR, Davis JM, Steer C, et al. Maternal seafood consumption in pregnancy and neurodevelopmental outcomes in childhood (ALSPAC study): an observational cohort study. *Lancet* 2007; 369(9561): 578–585.

Hornstra, G. Essential fatty acids in mothers and their neonates. *Am J Clin Nutr* 2000;71(suppl):1262S–1269S.

Imhoff-Kunsch B, Stein AD, Martorell R, et al. Prenatal docosahexaenoic acid supplementation and infant morbidity: randomized controlled trial. *Pediatrics* 2011 Sep 1;128(3):e505–e512.

Kohlboeck G, Glaser C, Tiesler C, et al. Effect of fatty acid status in cord blood serum on children's behavioral difficulties at 10 years of age: results from the LISAplus Study. *Am J Clin Nutr* 2011 Dec;94(6):1592–1599.

Koletzko et al. The roles of long-chain polyunsaturated fatty acids in pregnancy, lactation and infancy: review of current knowledge and consensus recommendations. *J Perinat Med* 2008;36:5–14.

Makrides M, Gibson RA, McPhee AJ, et al. Effect of DHA supplementation during pregnancy on maternal depression and neurodevelopment of young children: a randomized controlled trial. *JAMA* 2010 Oct 20;304(15):1675–1683.

Noakes PS, Vlachava M, Kremmyda LS, et al. Increased intake of oily fish in pregnancy: effects on neonatal immune responses and on clinical outcomes in infants at 6 mo. *Am J Clin Nutr* 2012 Feb;95(2):395–404.

Oken E, et al. Associations of maternal fish intake during pregnancy and breastfeeding duration with attainment of developmental milestones in early childhood: a study from the Danish National Birth Cohort. *Am J Clin Nutr* 2008 Sep;88(3):789–796.

Rondanelli M, Giacosa A, Opizzi A, et al. Effect of omega-3 fatty acids supplementation on depressive symptoms and on health-related quality of life in the treatment of elderly women with depression: a double-blind, placebo-controlled, randomized clinical trial. *J Am Coll Nutr* 2010; 29(1): 55–64.

Skilton MR, Ayer JG, Harmer JA, et al. Impaired fetal growth and arterial wall thickening: a randomized trial of omega-3 supplementation. *Pediatrics* 2012 Feb 20. [Epub ahead of print]

Stinson AM, Wiegand RD, Anderson RE. Recycling of docosahexaenoic acid in rat retinas during n-3 fatty acid deficiency. *J Lipid Res* 1991 Dec; 32(12): 2009–2017.

Chapter 11

Crowe FL, Skeaff CM, Green TJ, et al. Serum phospholipid n–3 long-chain polyunsaturated fatty acids and physical and mental health in a population-based survey of New Zealand adolescents and adults. *AJCN* Nov 2007; 86(5): 1278–1285.

Dullemeijer C, Durga J, Brouwer IA, et al. N–3 fatty acid proportions in plasma and cognitive performance in older adults. *AJCN* Nov 2007; 86(5): 1479–1485.

Gamoh S, Hashimoto M, Sugioka K, et al. Chronic administration of docosahexaenoic acid improves reference memory-related learning ability in young rats. *Neuroscience* 1999;93:237– 241.

Gao Q, Niti M, Feng L, et al. Omega-3 polyunsaturated fatty acid supplements and cognitive decline: Singapore Longitudinal Aging Studies. *J Nutr Health Aging* 2011; 15(1): 32–35.

Helland IB, Smith L, Saarem K, et al. Maternel supplementation with very-long-chain n-3 fatty acids during pregnancy and lactation augments children's IQ at 4 years of age. *Pediatrics* 2003;111:39–44.

Kim JL, Winkvist A, Aberg MA, et al. Fish consumption and school grades in Swedish adolescents: a study of the large general population. *Acta Paediatr* 2010; 99(1): 72–77.

McGahon BM, Martin DS, Horrobin DF, et al. Age-related changes in synaptic function: analysis of the effect of dietary supplementation with omega-3 fatty acids. *Neuroscience* 1999;94:305–314.

Milte CM, Sinn N, Street SJ, et al. Erythrocyte polyunsaturated fatty acid status, memory, cognition and mood in older adults with mild cognitive impairment and healthy controls. *Prostaglandins Leukot Essent Fatty Acids* 2011 May–Jun; 84(5–6): 153–1561.

Morris MC, Evans DA, Tangney CC, et al. Fish consumption and cognitive decline with age in a large community study. *Arch Neurol* 2005; 62: 1849–1853.

Muldoon MF, Ryan CM, Sheu L, et al. Serum phospholipid docosahexaenoic acid is associated with cognitive functioning during middle adulthood. *J Nutr* 2010 Apr; 140(4): 848–853.

Newman PE. Alzheimer's disease revisited. *Med Hypotheses* 2000;54:774–776.

Nurk E, Drevon CA, Refsum R, et al. Cognitive performance among the elderly and dietary fish intake: the Hordaland Health Study. *AJCN* Nov 2007; 86(5): 1470-1478.

Oken E, Wright RO, Kleinman KP, et al. Maternal fish consumption, hair mercury, and infant cognition in a U.S. cohort. *Environ Health Perspect* 2005 Oct; 113(10):1376–1380.

Sinn N, Milte CM, Street SJ, et al. Effects of n-3 fatty acids, EPA v. DHA, on depressive symptoms, quality of life, memory and executive function in older adults with mild cognitive impairment: a 6-month randomised controlled trial. *Br J Nutr* 2011 Sep 20:1–12.

Van Gelder BM, Tijhuis M, Kalmijn S, et al. Fish consumption, n-3 fatty acids, and subsequent 5-y cognitive decline in elderly men: the Zutphen Elderly Study. *AJCN* 2007 Apr; 85(4):1142–1147.

Whalley LK, et al. N-3 fatty acid erythrocyte membrane content, APOE varepsilon4, and cognitive variation: an observational follow-up study in late adulthood, *AJCN* 2008;87(2):449–454.

Yurko-Mauro K, McCarthy D, Rom D, et al. Beneficial effects of docosahexaenoic acid on cognition in age-related cognitive decline. *Alzheimers Dement* 2010 Nov;6(6): 456–464.

Chapter 12

Barberger-Gateau P, Raffaitin C, Letenneur L, et al. Dietary patterns and risk of dementia: the Three-City Cohort study. *Neurology* 2007;69(20):1921–1930.

Bazan NG. Neuroprotectin D1 (NPD1): a DHA-derived mediator that protects brain and retina against cell injury-induced oxidative stress. *Brain Pathol* 2005;15:159–166.

Bowman GL, Silbert LC, Howieson D, et al. Nutrient biomarker patterns, cognitive function, and MRI measures of brain aging. *Neurology* 2012 Jan 24;78(4):241–249.

Chiu CC, Frangou S, Chang CJ, et al. Associations between n-3 PUFA concentrations and cognitive function after recovery from late-life depression. *Am J Clin Nutr* 2012 Jan 4. [Epub ahead of print]

Freund-Levi Y, Eriksdotter-Jonhagen M, Cederholm T, et al. Omega-3 fatty acid treatment in 174 patients with mild to moderate Alzheimer disease—OmegAD study: a randomized double-blind trial. *Arch Neurol* 2006 Oct;63(10):1402–1408.

Freund-Levi Y, Hjorth E, Lindberg C, et al. Effects of omega-3 fatty acids on inflammatory markers in cerebrospinal fluid and plasma in Alzheimer's disease: the OmegAD study. *Dement Geriatr Cogn Disord* 2009;27(5):481–490.

GY Y, Schupf N, Cosentino SA, et al. Nutrient intake and plasma ß-amyloid. *Neurology* 2012 May 2 [Epub ahead of print].

Hamazaki T, Sawazaki S, Itomura M, et al. The effect of docosahexaenoic acid on aggression in young adults: a placebo-controlled double-blind study. *J Clin Invest* 1996;97:1129–1132.

Huang TL, Zandi PP, Tucker KL, et al. Benefits of fatty fish on dementia risk are stronger for those without APOE4. *Neurology* 2005;65(9):1409–1414.

Jicha GA, Markesbery WR. Omega-3 fatty acids: potential role in the management of early Alzheimer's disease. *Clin Interv Aging* 2010 Apr 7;5:45–61.

Kalmijn S, Launer LJ, Ott A. et al. Dietary fat intake and the risk of incident dementia in the Rotterdam Study. *Ann Neurol* 1997;42(5):776–782.

Kesse-Guyot E, Péneau S, Ferry M, et al. Thirteen-year prospective study between fish consumption, long-chain n-3 fatty acids intakes and cognitive function. *J Nutr Health Aging* 2011 Feb;15(2):115–120.

Ma QL, Teter B, Ubeda, OJ, et al. Omega-3 fatty acid docosahexaenoic acid increases SorLA/LR11, a sorting protein with reduced expression in sporadic Alzheimer's disease (AD): relevance to AD prevention. *J Neurosci* 2007;27:14299–14307.

Morris MC, Evans DA, Bienias JL, et al. Consumption of fish and n-3 fatty acids and risk of incident Alzheimer disease. *Arch Neurol* 2003;60(7):940–946.

Morris MC, Evans DA, Tangney CC, et al. Fish consumption and cognitive decline with age in a large community study. *Arch Neurol* 2005;62(12):1849–1853.

Quinn JF, Raman R, Thomas RG, et al. Docosahexaenoic acid supplementation and cognitive decline in Alzheimer disease: a randomized trial. *JAMA* 2010 Nov 3;304(17):1903–1911.

Raji C, Erickson K, Lopez O, et al. Regular fish consumption is associated with larger gray matter volumes and reduced risk for cognitive decline in the Cardiovascular Health Study. Paper presented at the annual meeting of the Radiological Society of North America, Dec 2 2011.

Schaefer EJ, Bongard V, Beiser AS, et al. Plasma phosphatidylcholine docosahexaenoic acid content and risk of dementia and Alzheimer disease: the Framingham Heart Study. *Arch Neurol* 2006;63(11):1545–1550.

Sinn N, Milte CM, Street SJ, et al. Effects of n-3 fatty acids, EPA v. DHA, on depressive symptoms, quality of life, memory and executive function in older adults with mild cognitive impairment: a 6-month randomised controlled trial. *Br J Nutr* 2011 Sep 20:1–12.

Tully AM, Roche HM, Doyle R, et al. Low serum cholesteryl ester-docosahexaenoic acid levels in Alzheimer's disease: a case-control study. *Br J Nutr* 2003;89(4):483–489.

Whalley LJ, Deary IJ, Starr JM, et al. N-3 Fatty acid erythrocyte membrane content, APOE varepsilon4, and cognitive variation: an observational follow-up study in late adulthood. *Am J Clin Nutr* 2008;87(2):449–454.

Yurko-Mauro K, McCarthy D, Rom D, et al. Beneficial effects of docosahexaenoic acid on cognition in age-related cognitive decline. *Alzheimers Dement* 2010 Nov;6(6): 456–464.

Zhao Y, Calon F, Julien C, et al. Docosahexaenoic acid-derived neuroprotectin D1 induces neuronal survival via secretase- and PPAR?-mediated mechanisms in Alzheimer's disease models. *PLoS One* 2011 Jan 5;6(1):e15816.

Chapter 13

Alexopoulos GS, Meyers BS, Young RC, et al. 'Vascular depression' hypothesis. *Arch Gen Psychiatry* 1997;54:915–922.

Andrade L, Caraveo-A. Epidemiology of major depressive episodes: results from the International Consortium of Psychiatric Epidemiology (ICPE) surveys. *Int J Methods Psychiatr Res* 2003;12(1):3–21.

Appleton KM, Rogers PI, Ness AR. Is there a role for n-3 long-chain polyunsaturated fatty acids in the regulation of mood and behaviour? A review of the evidence to date from epidemiological studies, clinical studies and intervention trials. *Nutr Res Rev* 2008 Jun;21(1):13–41.

Appleton KM, Rogers PI, Ness AR. Updated systematic review and meta-analysis of the effects of n-3 long-chain polyunsaturated fatty acids on depressed mood. *Amer J Clin Nutr* 2010 Mar; 91(3):757–770.

Australian Institute of Health and Welfare. National health priority areas report—mental health: a report focusing on depression, 1998. Available online at: www.health.gov.au/internet/main/publishing.nsf/content/8E0E3BC67E3962AFCA25712B0080235F/$File/nhpaall.pdf.

Buydens-Branchey L, Branchey M, Hibbeln, JR. Associations between increases in plasma n-3 polyunsaturated fatty acids following supplementation and decreases in anger and anxiety in substance abusers. *Prog Neuropsychopharmacol Biol Pyschiatry* 2008 Feb 15;32(2):568–575.

Chiu CC, Frangou S, Chang CJ, et al. Associations between n?3 PUFA concentrations and cognitive function after recovery from late-life depression. *Am J Clin Nutr* 2012 Feb; 95(2):420-407.

Crowe FL, Skeaff CM, Green TJ, et al. Serum phospholipid n-3 long-chain polyunsaturated fatty acids and physical and mental health in a population-based survey of New Zealand adolescents and adults. *J Clin Nutr* 2007 Nov;86(5):1278–1285.

Eaton WW, Anthony JC, Gallo J. Natural history of diagnostic interview schedule/DSM-IV major depression: the Baltimore Epidemiologic Catchment Area follow-up. *Arch Gen Psychiatry* 1997;54(11):993–999.

Edwards R, Peet M, Shay J, et al. Omega-3 polyunsaturated fatty acid levels in the diet and in red blood cell membranes of depressed patients. *J Affect Disord* 1998 Mar;48(2–3):149–155.

Fontani G, Corradeschi F, Felici A, et al. Cognitive and physiological effects of omega-3 polyunsaturated fatty acid supplementation in healthy subjects. *Eur J Clin Invest* 2005 Nov;35(11):691–699.

Fontani G, Lodi L, Migliorini S, et al. Effect of omega-3 and policosanol supplementation on attention and reactivity in athletes. *J Am Coll Nutr* 2009 Aug;28 suppl:473S–481S.

Freeman MP, Hibbeln, JR, Wisner KL, et al. Omega-3 fatty acids: evidence basis for treatment and future research in psychiatry. *J Clin Psychiatry* 2006;67:1954–1967.

Gesch CB, Hammond SM, Hampson SE, et al. Influence of supplementary vitamins, minerals and essential fatty acids on the antisocial behaviour of young adult prisoners: a randomised, placebo-controlled trial. *Br J Psychiatry* 2002;181: 22–28.

Giltay EJ, Geleijnse JM, Kromhout D. Effects of n23 fatty acids on depressive symptoms and dispositional optimism after myocardial infarction. *Am J Clin Nutr* 2011 Dec;94(6):1442–1450.

Hibbeln JR. Fish consumption and major depression. *Lancet* 1998 Apr 18;351(9110):1213.

Hibbeln JR, Salem N Jr. Dietary polyunsaturated fatty acids and depression: when cholesterol does not satisfy. *Am J Clin Nutr* 1995;62:1–9.

Hoffmire CA, Block RC, Thevenet-Morrison K, et al. Associations between omega-3 poly-unsaturated fatty acids from fish consumption and severity of depressive symptoms: an analysis of the 2005–2008 National Health and Nutrition Examination survey. *Prostag Leukotr Ess* 2012 Apr 3. [Epub ahead of print]

Jazayeri S, Tehrani-Doost M, Keshavar SA, et al. Comparison of therapeutic effects of omega-3 fatty acid eicosapentaenoic acid and fluoxetine, separately and in combination, in major depressive disorder. *Aust NZ J Psychiatry* 2008 Mar;42(3):192–198.

Kessler RC, Berglund P, Demler O, et al. Lifetime prevalence and age-of-onset distributions of DSM-IV disorders in the National Comorbidity Survey Replication. *Arch Gen Psychiatry* 2005;62(6):593–602.

Kessler RC, Berglund P, Demler O. The epidemiology of major depressive disorder: results from the National Comorbidity Survey Replication (NCS-R). *JAMA* 2003;289(203):3095–3105.

Klerman GL, Weissman MM. Increasing rates of depression. *JAMA* 1989;261(15): 2229–2235.

Kuehner C. Gender differences in unipolar depression: an update of epidemiological findings and possible explanations. *Acta Psychiatrica Scandinavica* 2003;108(3):163–174.

Lucas M, Asselin G, Mérette C, et al. Ethyl-eicosapentaenoic acid for the treatment of psychological distress and depressive symptoms in middle-aged women: a double-blind, placebo-controlled, randomized clinical trial. *Am J Clin Nutr* 2009 Feb;89(2):641–651.

Maes M, Smith R, Christophe A, et al. Fatty acid composition in major depression: decreased omega 3 fractions in cholesteryl esters and increased C20:4 omega 6/C20:5 omega 3 ratio in cholesteryl esters and phospholipids. *J Affect Disord* 1996;38:35–46.

Maes M. Major depression and activation of the inflammatory response system. In: *Cytokines, Stress, and Depression* edited by R Dantzer R, EE Wollman EE, R Yirmiya R. New York: Kluwer Academic/Plenum Publishers, 1999.

Mathers CD, Loncar D. Updated projections of global mortality and burden of disease, 2002–2030: data sources, methods and results. Geneva, Switzerland: WHO, 2005.

McNamara RK, Hahn CG, Jandacek R, et al., Selective defects in the omega-3 fatty acid docosahexaenoic acid in the postmortem orbitofrontal cortex of patients with major depressive disorder. *Biol Psychiatry* 2007;62(1):17–24.

Miranda J, Duan N, Sherbourn CD, et al. The societal promise of improving care for depression, 2008. Available online at: www.rand.org/pubs/research_briefs/RB9055-1.html.

Mischoulon, D. The impact of omega-3 fatty acids on depressive orders and suicidality. *J Clin Psychiatry* 2011 Dec;72(12):1574–1576.

Mullen BJ, Martin RJ. The effect of dietary fat on diet selection may involve central serotonin. *Am J Physiol* 1992;263:R559–63.

Murphy JM, Laird NM, Monson RR, et al. A 40-year perspective on the prevalence of depression: the Stirling County study. *Arch Gen Psychiatry* 2000;57(3):209–215.

Pottala JV, Talley JA, Churchill SW, et al. Red blood cell fatty acids are associated with depression in a case-control study of adolescents. *Prostag Leukotr Ess* 2012 Apr 5. [Epub ahead of print]

Rondanelli M, Giacosa A, Opizzi A, et al. Effect of omega-3 fatty acids supplementation on depressive symptoms and on health-related quality of life in the treatment of elderly women with depression: a double-blind, placebo-controlled, randomized clinical trial. *J Amer Coll Nutr* 2010 Feb;29(1):55–64.

Rudin DO, Felix C. *Omega-3 Oils.* Honesdale, PA: Paragon Press, 1996.

Salem N Jr, Litman B, Kim HY, et al. Mechanisms of action of docosahexaenoic acid in the nervous system. *Lipids* 2001;36:945–959.

Salem N Jr, Shingu T, Kim HY, et al. Specialization in membrane structure and metabolism with respect to polyunsaturated lipids. *Prog Clin Biol Res* 1988;282:319–333.

Schoenstadt A. Depression statistics. *MedTV* 2008. Available online at: www. depression. emedtv.com/depression/depression-statistics.html.

Severus, WE, Ahrens B, Stoll AL. Omega-3 fatty acids: the missing link? *Arch Gen Psychiatry* 1999 Apr;56(4):380–381.

Silvers KM, Scott KM. Fish consumption and self-reported physical and mental health status. *Public Health Nutr* 2002;5:427–431.

Smith RS. The macrophage theory of depression. *Medical Hypothesis* 1991;35:298–306.

Stoll AL, et al. Omega-3 fatty acids in bipolar disorder: a preliminary double-blind, placebo-controlled trial. *Arch Gen Psychiatry* 1999;56:407–412.

Sublette ME, Ellis SP, Geant AL, et al. Meta-analysis of the effects of eicosapentaenoic acid (EPA) in clinical trials in depression. *J Clin Psychiatry* 2011 Dec;72(12):1577–1584.

Tiemeier H, van Tuijl HR, Hofman A, et al. Plasma fatty acid composition and depression are associated in the elderly: the Rotterdam Study. *Am J Clin Nutr* 2003 Jul;78(1):40–46.

Weissman MM, Wickramaratne P, Greenwald S, et al. The changing rate of major depression. *JAMA* 1992;268:3098–3105.

World Health Organization. The world health report 2001—mental health: new understanding, new hope. Available online at: www.who.int/whr/2001/en.

Zaalberg A, Nijiman H, Bulten E, et al. Effects of nutritional supplements on aggression, rule-breaking, and psychopathology among young adult prisoners. *Aggress Behav* 2010 Mar-Apr;36(2):117–126.

Chapter 14

Akter K, Gallo DA, Martin SA, et al. A review of the possible role of the essential fatty acids and fish oils in the aetiology, prevention or pharmacotherapy of schizophrenia. *J Clin Pharm Ther* 2011 Apr;37(2):132–139.

Amminger GP, Schäfer MR, Papageorgiou K, et al. Long-chain omega-3 fatty acids for indicated prevention of psychotic disorders: a randomized, placebo-controlled trial. *Arch Gen Psychiatry* 2010 Feb;67(2):146–154.

Assies J, Lieverse R, Vreken P, et al. Significantly reduced docosahexaenoic and docosapentaenoic acid concentrations in erythrocyte membranes from schizophrenic patients compared with a carefully matched control group. *Biol Psychiatry* 2001 Mar 15;49(6):510–522.

Bostwick JM, Pankratz VS. Affective disorders and suicide risk: a reexamination. *Am J Psychiatry* 2000;157:1925–1932.

Chiu CC, Huang SY, Su KP, et al. Polyunsaturated fatty acid deficit in patients with bipolar mania. *Eur Neuropsychopharmacol* 2003;13:99–103.

Clayton EH, Hanstock TL, Hirneth SJ, et al. Reduced mania and depression in juvenile bipolar disorder associated with long-chain omega-3 polyunsaturated fatty acid supplementation. *Eur J Clin Nutr* 2009;63(8):1037–1040.

Emsley R, Myburgh C, Oosthuizen P, et al. Randomized, placebo-controlled study of ethyl-eicosapentaenoic acid as supplemental treatment in schizophrenia. *Amer J Psychiatry* 2002 Sep;159(9):1596–1598.

Frangou S, Lewis M, McCrone P. Efficacy of ethyl-eicosapentaenoic acid in bipolar depression: randomised double-blind placebo-controlled study. *Br J Psychiatry* 2006; 188:46–50.

Hale RS. Omega-3 study approved in Iraq. US Army 2010 Sept. Available online at: www.army.mil/article/45778/Omega_3_study_approved_in_Iraq.

Huan M, Hamazaki K, Sun Y, et al. Suicide attempt and n-3 fatty acid levels in red blood cells: a case control study in China. *Biological Psychiatry* 2004;56(7):490–496.

Judd LL, Akiskal HS. The prevalence and disability of bipolar spectrum disorders in the US population: re-analysis of the ECA database taking into account subthreshold cases. *J Affect Disord* 2003;73:123–131.

Lewis MD, Hibbeln JR, Johnson JE, et al. Suicide deaths of active-duty US military and omega-3 fatty-acid atatus: a case-control comparison. *J Clin Psychiatry* 2011 Aug 23. [Epub ahead of print]

Mischoulon D, Papakostas GI, Dording CM, et al. A double-blind, randomized controlled trial of ethyl-eicosapentaenoate for major depressive disorder. *J Clin Psychiatry* 2009 Dec;70(12): 1636–1644.

Noaghiul S, Hibbeln JR. Cross-national comparisons of seafood consumption and rates of bipolar disorders. *Am J Psychiatry* 2003;160:2222–2227.

Peet M, Brind J, Ramschand CN, et al. Two double-blind placebo-controlled pilot studies of eicosapentaenoic acid in the treatment of schizophrenia. *Schizophenr Res* 2001 Apr 30;49(3):243–251.

Peet M, Stokes C. Omega-3 fatty acids in the treatment of psychiatric disorders. *Drugs* 2005;65(8):1051–1059.

Ranjekar PK, Hinge A, Hegde MV, et al. Decreased antioxidant enzymes and membrane essential polyunsaturated fatty acids in schizophrenic and bipolar mood disorder patients. *Psychiatry Res* 2003;121:109–122.

Stoll AL, Severus WE, Freeman MP, et al. Omega 3 fatty acids in bipolar disorder: a preliminary double-blind, placebo-controlled trial. *Arch Gen Psychiatry* 1999;56: 407–412.

Tartakovsky M. Schizophrenia fact sheet. PsychCentral.com 2012 Mar. Available online at: psychcentral.com/lib/2009/schizophrenia-fact-sheet.

Wu EQ, Birnbaum HG, Shi L, et al. The economic burden of schizophrenia in the United States in 2002. *J Clin Psychiatry* 2005 Sep;66(9):1122–1129.

Chapter 15

Augood C, Chakravarthy U, Young I, et al. Oily fish consumption, dietary docosahexaenoic acid and eicosapentaenoic acid intakes, and associations with neovascular age-related macular degeneration. *Am J Clin Nutr* 2008 Aug;88(2):398–406.

Birch EE, Carlson SE, Hoffman DR, et al. The DIAMOND study: a double-masked, randomized controlled clinical trial of the maturation of infant visual acuity as a function of the dietary level of docosahexaenoic acid. *Am J Clin Nutr* 2010 Apr; 91(4):848–859.

Brignole-Baudouin F, Baudouin C, Aragona P, et al. A multicentre, double-masked, randomized, controlled trial assessing the effect of oral supplementation of omega-3 and omega-6 fatty acids on a conjunctival inflammatory marker in dry eye patients. *Acta Ophthalmol* 2011 Nov;89(7):e591–e597.

Cakiner-Egilmez T. Omega 3 fatty acids and the eye. *Insight* 2008 Oct–Dec;33(4):20–25.

Christen WG, Schaumberg DA, Glynn RJ, et al. Dietary omega-3 fatty acid and fish intake and incident age-related macular degeneration in women." *Arch Ophthalmol* 2011; 129(7): 921–929.

Chua B, Flood B, Rochtchina E, et al. Dietary fatty acids and the 5-year incidence of age-related maculopathy. *Arch Ophthalmol* 2006 Jul;124(7):981–986.

Donoso LA, Kim D, Frost A, et al. The role of inflammation in the pathogenesis of age-related macular degeneration. *Surv Ophthalmol* 2006;51:137–152.

Friedman DS, O'Colmain BJ, Muñoz B, et al. Prevalence of age-related macular degeneration in the United States. *Arch Ophthalmol* 2004;122:564–572.

Jeffrey BG, Neuringer M. Age-related decline in rod phototransduction sensitivity in rhesus monkeys fed an n-3 fatty acid-deficient diet. *Invest Ophthalmol Vis Sci* 2009;50(9):4360–4367.

Li N, He J, Schwartz CE, et al. Resolvin E1 improves tear production and decreases inflammation in a dry eye mouse model. *J Ocul Pharmacol Ther* 2010 Oct;26(5):431–439.

Merle B, Delyfer MN, Korobelnik JF, et al. Dietary omega-3 fatty acids and the risk for age-related maculopathy: the Alienor study. *Invest Ophthalmol Vis Sci* 2011 Jul 29;52(8):6004-6011.

Moeller SM, Voland R, Tinker L, et al. Associations between age-related nuclear cataract and lutein and zeaxanthin in the diet and serum in the carotenoids in the Age-Related Eye Disease Study: an ancillary study of the Women's Health Initiative. *Arch Ophthalmol* 2008 Mar;126(3):354–364.

National Eye Institute. Facts about dry eye. National Institutes of Health, 2009 Aug. Avaialable online at: www.nei.nih.gov/health/dryeye/dryeye.asp#a.

National Eye Institute. Statistics and data. National Institutes of Health, 2004 Apr. Available online at: www.nei.nih.gov/eyedata/pbd_tables.asp.

Penfold PL, Madigan MC, Gillies MC, et al. Immunological and etiological aspects of macular degeneration. *Prog Retin Eye Res* 2001;20:385–414.

Rand AL, Asbell PA. Nutritional supplements for dry eye syndrome. *Curr Opin Ophthalmol* 2011 Jul;22(4):279–282.

Roncone M, Bartlett H, Eperjesi F. Essential fatty acids for dry eye: a review. *Cont Lens Anterior Eye* 2010 Apr;33(2):49–54.

SanGiovanni JP, Agrón E, Meleth AD, et al. Omega-3 long-chain polyunsaturated fatty acid intake and 12-y incidence of neovascular age-related macular degeneration and central geographic atrophy. *Am J Clin Nutr* 2009 Dec;90(6):1601–1607.

SanGiovanni JP, Chew EY, Agron E, et al. The relationship of dietary omega-3 long-chain polyunsaturated fatty acid intake with incident age-related macular degeneration: AREDS report no. 23. *Arch Ophthalmol* 2008 Sep;126(9):1274–1279.

Seddon JM, Cote J, Rosner B. Progression of age-related macular degeneration: association with dietary fat, transunsaturated fat, nuts, and fish intake. *Arch Ophthalmol* 2003;121(12):1728–1737.

Seddon JM, George S, Rosner B. Cigarette smoking, fish consumption, omega-3 fatty acid intake, and associations with age-related macular degeneration: the US Twin Study of age-related macular degeneration. *Arch Ophthalmol* 2006 Jul;124(7):995–1001.

Smith W, Mitchell P, Leeder SR. Dietary fat and fish intake and age-related maculopathy. *Arch Ophthalmol* 2000 Mar;118(3):401–404.

Stinson AM, Wiegand RD, Anderson RE. Recycling of docosahexaenoic acid in rat retinas during n-3 fatty acid deficiency. *J Lipid Res* 1991 Dec;32(12):2009–2017.

Wojtowicz JC, Butovich I, Uchiyama E, et al. Pilot, prospective, randomized, double-masked, placebo-controlled clinical trial of an omega-3 supplement for dry eye. *Cornea* 2011 Mar;30(3):308–314.

Chapter 16

Ahmad A, Banerjee S, Wang Z, et al. Aging and inflammation: etiological culprits of cancer. *Curr Aging Sci* 2009;2(3):174–186.

Armanios M, et al,. "Short telomeres are sufficient to cause the degenerative defects associated with aging," *Am J Hum Genet* 2009 Dec 11; 85(6):823–832.

Bakaysa SL, Mucci LA, Slagboom PE, et al. Telomere length predicts survival independent of genetic influences. *Aging Cell* 2007 Dec;6(6):769–774.

Campisi J. Senescent cells, tumor suppression, and organismal aging: good citizens, bad neighbors. *Cell* 2005 Feb 25;120(4):513–522.

Chan SR, Blackburn EH. Telomeres and telomerase. *Philos Trans R Soc Lond B Biol Sci* 2004;359(1441):109–121.

Crowe FL, et al., Serum phospholipid n-3 long-chain polyunsaturated fatty acids and physical and mental health in a population-based survey of New Zealand adolescents and adults. *Am J Clin Nutr* 2007;86(5):1278–1285.

Danaei G, Ding EL, Mozaffarian D, et al. The preventable causes of death in the United States: comparative risk assessment of dietary, lifestyle, and metabolic risk factors. *PLoS Med* 2009;6(4):e1000058.

De Spirt S, Stahl W, Tronnier, H, et al. Intervention with flaxseed and borage oil supplements modulates skin condition in women. *Br J Nutr* 2009 Feb;101(3):440–445.

Einvik G, Klemsdal TO, Sandvik L, et al. A randomized clinical trial on n-3 polyunsaturated fatty acids supplementation and all-cause mortality in elderly men at high cardiovascular risk. *Eur J Cardiovasc Prev Rehabil* 2010 Oct;17(5):588–592.

Farzaneh-Far R, et al. Association of marine omega-3 fatty acid levels with telomeric aging in patients with coronary heart disease. *JAMA* 2010;303(3):250–257.

Farzaneh-Far R. et al. Telomere length trajectory and its determinants in persons with coronary artery disease: longitudinal findings from the Heart and Soul Study. *PLoS One* 2010;5(1): e8612.

Fitzpatrick AL, Kronmal RA, Kimura M, et al. Leukocyte telomere length and mortality in the Cardiovascular Health Study. *J Gerontol A Biol Sci Med Sci* 2011 Apr;66(4):421–429.

Gopinath B, Buyken AE, Flood VM, et al. of polyunsaturated fatty acids, fish, and nuts and risk of inflammatory disease mortality. *Am J Clin Nutr* 2011 may;93(5):1073–1079.

Lindberg M, Saltvedt I, Sletvold O, et al. Long-chain n-3 fatty acids and mortality in elderly patients. *Am J Clin Nutr* 2008 Sep;88(3):722–729.

McCusker MM, Grant-Kels JM. Healing fats of the skin: the structural and immunologic roles of the omega-6 and omega-3 fatty acids. *Clin Dermatol* 2010 Jul-Aug;28(4):440–451.

Olovnikov AM. Telomeres, telomerase, and aging: origin of the theory. *Exp Gerontol* 1996;31(4):443–448.

Omer TN, Hsueh WC, Blackbur EH, et al. Association between telomere length, specific causes of death, and years of healthy life in health, aging, and body composition, a population-based cohort study," *J Gerontol A Biol Sci Med Sci* Aug 2009; 64A(8):860–864.

Pottala JV, Garg S, Cohen BE, et al. Eicosapentaenoic and docosahexaenoic acids predict all-cause mortality in patients with stable coronary heart disease: the Heart and Soul Study. *Circ Cardiovasc Qual Outcomes* 2010 Jul;3(4):406–412.

Romieu I, Garcia-Esteban R, Sunyer J, et al. The effect of supplementation with omega-3 polyunsaturated fatty acids on markers of oxidative stress in elderly exposed to PM(2.5). *Environ Health Perspect* 2008;116(9):1237–1242.

Chapter 17

American College of Rheumatology Subcommittee. Guidelines for the management of rheumatoid arthritis: 2002 Update. *Arthritis Rheum* 2002;46(2):328–346.

Boddaert J, Huong DL, Amoura Z, et al. Late-onset systemic lupus erythematosus: a personal series of 47 patients and pooled analysis of 714 cases in the literature. *Medicine* (Baltimore). Nov 2004;83(6):348–359.

Buckwalter JA, Saltzman C, Brown T. The impact of osteoarthritis. *Clin Orthoped Rel Res* 2004:427S:S6–S15.

Calder PC. Session 3: Joint Nutrition Society and Irish Nutrition and Dietetic Institute Symposium on Nutrition and autoimmune disease PUFA, inflammatory processes and rheumatoid arthritis. *Proc Nutr Soc* 2008 Nov;67(4):409–418.

Calder PC. The scientific basis for fish oil supplementation in rheumatoid arthritis. In: Ransley JK, Donnelly JK, Read NW, eds. *Nutritional Supplements in Health and Disease.* London, United Kingdom: Springer Verlag, 2001:175–197.

Calder PC, Zurier RB. Polyunsaturated fatty acids and rheumatoid arthritis. *Curr Opin Clin Nutr Metab Care* 2001;4:115–121.

Cleland LG, et al. Reduction of cardiovascular risk factors with longterm fish oil treatment in early rheumatoid arthritis. *J Rheumatol* 2006 Oct;33(10):1973–1979.

Cleland LG, Caughey GE, James MJ, et al. Reduction of cardiovascular risk factors with longterm fish oil treatment in early rheumatoid arthritis. *J Rheumatol* 2006;33: 1973–1979.

Cleland LG, James MJ. Fish oil and rheumatoid arthritis: anti-inflammatory and collateral health benefits. *J Rheumatol* 2000;27:2305–2307.

Cleland LG, James MJ. Fish oil for anti-inflammatory effect: a practical approach to symptom control with reduced risk. *PUFA Newsletter* 2006 Dec. Available online at: www.fatsoflife.com/article.php?nid=1&edition=arch&id=392&issueid=50.

Cleland LG, James MJ, Proudman SM. Dietary fats and inflammation: the medicinal use of fish oil. *Nutrition & Dietetics* 2009;66:4–6.

Cleland LG, James MJ, Proudman SM. Fish oil: what the prescriber needs to know. *Arthritis Res Ther* 2006;8(1):202.

Cleland LG, James MJ, Proudman SM. The role of fish oils in the treatment of rheumatoid arthritis. *Drugs* 2003;63:845–853.

Gabriel SE, Crowson CS, Campion ME, et al. Direct medical costs unique to people with arthritis. *J Rheumatol* 1997;24(4):719–725.

Gabriel SE, Crowson CS, Luthra HS, et al. Modeling the lifetime costs of rheumatoid arthritis. *J Rheumatol* 1999;26(6):1269–1274.

Gabriel SE, Crowson CS, O'Fallon WM. The epidemiology of rheumatoid arthritis in Rochester, Minnesota, 1955–1985. *Arthritis Rheum* 1999;42(3):415–420.

Galarraga B, Ho M, Youssef HM, et al. Cod liver oil (n-3 fatty acids) as a non-steroidal anti-inflammatory drug sparing agent in rheumatoid arthritis. *Rheumatology* (Oxford). 2008;47(5):665–669.

Geusens PP. N–3 fatty acids in the treatment of rheumatoid arthritis. In: Kremer JM, ed. *Medicinal Fatty Acids in Inflammation*. Basel, Switzerland: Birkhauser Verlag, 1998.

Gingras AA, White PJ, Chouinard PY, et al., Long-chain omega-3 fatty acids regulate bovine whole-body protein metabolism by promoting muscle insulin signaling to the Akt-mTOR-S6K1 pathway and insulin sensitivity. *J Physiol* 2007 Feb 15;579(Pt 1):269–284.

Goldberg RJ, Katz J. A meta-analysis of the analgesic effects of omega-3 polyunsaturated fatty acid supplementation on 823 patients for inflammatory joint pain. *Pain* 2007;129:210–223.

Helmick CG, Felson DT, Lawrence RC, et al. Estimates of the prevalence of arthritis and other rheumatic conditions in the United States. Part I. *Arthritis Rheum* Jan 2008;58(1):15–25.

James MJ, Cleland LG. Dietary n–3 fatty acids and therapy for rheumatoid arthritis. *Semin Arthritis Rheum* 1997;27:85–97.

Jump DB. N-3 polyunsaturated fatty acid regulation of hepatic gene transcription. *Curr Opin Lipidol* 2008 Jun;19(3):242–247.

Klein-Gitelman M, Reiff A, Silverman ED. Systemic lupus erythematosus in childhood. *Rheum Dis Clin North Am* Aug 2002;28(3):561–577.

Kremer JM. N–3 fatty acid supplements in rheumatoid arthritis. *Am J Clin Nutr* 2000;71(suppl):349S–3451S.

Lawrence RC, Felson DT, Helmick CG, et al. Estimates of the prevalence of arthritis and other rheumatic conditions in the United States. Part II. *Arthritis Rheum* 2008; 58(1):26–35.

Maetzel A, Li LC, Pencharz J, et al. The economic burden associated with osteoarthritis, rheumatoid arthritis, and hypertension: a comparative study. *Ann Rheum Dis* 2004;63(4):395–401.

Makhoul Z, Kristal AR, Gulati R, et al. Associations of very high intakes of eicosapentaenoic and docosahexaenoic acids with biomarkers of chronic disease risk among Yup'ik Eskimos. *Am J Clin Nutr* 2010;91(3):777–785.

Manzi S. Epidemiology of systemic lupus erythematosus. *Am J Manag Care* Oct 2001;7(16 suppl):S474–S479.

Maradit-Kremers H, Nicola PJ, Crowson CS, et al. Cardiovascular death in rheumatoid arthritis: A population-based study. *Arthritis Rheum* 2005;52:722–732.

Recht L, Helin P, Rasmussen JO, et al. Hand handicap and rheumatoid arthritis in a fish-eating society: the Faroe Islands. *J Intern Med* 1990 Jan;227(1):49–55.

Reinders I, et al. Association of serum n-3 polyunsaturated fatty acids with C-reactive protein in men. *Eur J Clin Nutr* 2011 Nov 23. doi: 10.1038/ejcn.2011.195. [Epub ahead of print]).

Rodacki CL, Rodacki AL, Pereira G, et al. Fish-oil supplementation enhances the effects of strength training in elderly women. *Am J Clin Nutr* 2012 Jan 4. [Epub ahead of print]

Smith GI, Atherton P, Reeds DN, et al. Dietary omega-3 fatty acid supplementation increases the rate of muscle protein synthesis in older adults: a randomized controlled trial. *Am J Clin Nutr* Feb2011;93(2):402–412.

Volker D, Garg M. Dietary n–3 fatty acid supplementation in rheumatoid arthritis— mechanisms, clinical outcomes, controversies, and future directions. *J Clin Biochem Nutr* 1996;20:83–87.

Chapter 18

Aronson WJ, et al. Phase II Prospective Randomized Trial of a Low-Fat Diet with Fish Oil Supplementation in Men Undergoing Radical Prostatectomy. *Cancer Prev Res* 2011 Dec;4(12):2062–2071.

Berquin IM, Edwards IJ, Chen YQ. Multi-targeted therapy of cancer by omega-3 fatty acids. *Cancer Lett* 2008;269:363–377.

Boyer BB, Mohatt GV, Plaetke R, et al. Metabolic syndrome in Yup'ik Eskimos: the Center for Alaska Native Health Research (CANHR) Study. *Obesity* 2007;15(11): 2535–2540.

Browning LM, Krebs JK, Moore CS, et al. The impact of long chain n-3 polyunsaturated fatty acid supplementation on inflammation, insulin sensitivity and CVD risk in a group of overweight women with an inflammatory phenotype. *Diabetes Obes Metab* 2007;9:70–80.

De Caterina R, Madonna R, Bertolotto A, et al. n-3 fatty acids in the treatment of diabetic patients: biological rationale and clinical data. *Diabetes Care* 2007 Apr;30(4):1012–1026.

Derosa G, Cicero AFG, Fogari E, et al. Effects of n-3 PUFA on insulin resistance after an oral fat load. *European Journal of Lipid Science and Technology* Published online ahead of print, doi: 10.1002/ejlt.201000504)

Djoussé L, Biggs ML, Lemaitre RN, et al. Plasma omega-3 fatty acids and incident diabetes in older adults. *Amer J Clin Nutr* 2011 Aug: 94)2):527–533.

Ebbesson SO, Risica PM, Ebbesson LO, et al. Omega-3 fatty acids improve glucose tolerance and components of the metabolic syndrome in Alaskan Eskimos: the Alaska Siberia project. *Int J Circumpolar Health* 2005;64(4):396–408.

Fedor D, Kelley DS. Prevention of insulin resistance by n-3 polyunsaturated fatty acids. *Curr Opin Clin Nutr Metab Care* 2009 Mar;12(2):138–146.

Feskens EJM, Loeber JG, Kromhout D. Diet and physical activity as determinants of hyperinsulinemia: the Zutphen Elderly Study. *Am J Epidemiol* 1994;140:350–360.

Ginsberg HN, Illingworth DR. Postprandial dyslipidemia: an atherogenic disorder common in patients with diabetes mellitus. *Am J Cardiol* 2001;88(6A):9H–15H.

Gleissman H. et al. Docosahexaenoic acid metabolome in neural tumors: identification of cytotoxic intermediates. *FASEB Journal* 2010;24:906–915.

Haag M, Dippenaar NG. Dietary fats, fatty acids and insulin resistance: short review of a multifaceted connection. *Med Sci Monit* 2005;11(12):RA359–RA367.

Knight JA, Lesosky M, Barnett H, et al. Vitamin D and reduced risk of breast cancer: a population-based case-control study. *Cancer Epidemiol Biomarkers Prev* 2007;16: 422–429.

Larsson SC, Kumlin M, Ingelman-Sundberg M, et al. Dietary long-chain n-3 fatty acids for the prevention of cancer: a review of potential mechanisms. *Am J Clin Nutr* 2004;79:935–945.

Lopez-Alarcón M, et al. Supplementation of n-3 long-chain polyunsaturated fatty acid synergistically decreases insulin resistance with weight loss of obese prepubertal and pubertal children. *Arch Med Res* 2011 Aug;42(6):502–508.

Martín de Santa Olalla L, Sánchez Muniz FJ, Vaquero MP. N-3 fatty acids in glucose metabolism and insulin sensitivity. *Nutr Hosp* 2009 Mar-Apr;24(2):113–127.

Menzaghi C, Trischitta V, Doria A. Genetic influences of adiponectin on insulin resistance, type 2 diabetes, and cardiovascular disease. *Diabetes* 2007;56:1198–1209.

Nettleton JA, Katz J. N-3 long-chain polyunsaturated fatty acids in type 2 diabetes: a review. *Amer Diet Assoc* 2005 Mar;105(3):428–440.

Norris JM, Yin X, Lamb MM, et al. Omega-3 polyunsaturated fatty acid intake and islet autoimmunity in children at increased risk for type 1 diabetes. *JAMA* 2007;298(12):1420–1428.

Oliver E, McGillicuddy F, et al. The role of inflammation and macrophage accumulation in the development of obesity-induced type 2 diabetes mellitus and the possible therapeutic effects of long-chain n-3PUFA. *Proc Nutr Soc* 2010;69(2):232–243.

Rudkowska I. Fish oils for cardiovascular disease: impact on diabetes. *Maturitas* 2010 Sep;67(1):25–28.

Saadatian-Elahi M, Norat T, Goudable J, et al. Biomarkers of dietary fatty acid intake and the risk of breast cancer: a meta-analysis. *Int J Cancer* 2004;111:584–591.

Sirtori CR, Galli C. N-3 fatty acids and diabetes. *Biomed Pharmacother* 2002 Oct; 56(8):397–406.

Stene LC, Joner G, Norwegian Childhood Diabetes Study Group. Use of cod liver oil during the first year of life is associated with lower risk of childhood-onset type 1 diabetes: a large, population-based, case-control study. *Am J Clin Nutr* 2003 Dec;78(6): 1128–1134.

Stirban A, Nandrean S, Götting C, et al. Effects of n-3 fatty acids on macro- and micro-vascular function in subjects with type 2 diabetes mellitus. *Amer J Clin Nutr* 2010 Mar;91(3):808–813.

Storlien LH, Jenkins AB, Chisholm DJ, et al. Influence of dietary fat composition on development of insulin resistance in rats: relationship to muscle triglyceride and omega-3 fatty acids in muscle phospholipid. *Diabetes* 1991 Feb;40(2):280–289.

Thorsdottir I, Hill J, Ramel A. Omega-3 fatty acid supply from milk associates with lower type 2 diabetes in men and coronary heart disease in women. *Prev Med* 2004;39:630–634.

Vilgbersson S, Sigurdsson G, Sigvaldason H, et al. Prevalence and incidence of NIDDM in Iceland: evidence for stable incidence among males and females 1967–1991—the Reikjavik Study. *Diabet Med* 1997;14:491–498.

Villegas R, Xiang YB, Elasy T, et al. Fish, shellfish, and long-chain n-3 fatty acid consumption and risk of incident type 2 diabetes in middle-aged Chinese men and women. *Am J Clin Nutr* 2011 Jun 15. [Epub ahead of print]

Wu JH, Lemaitre RN, King IB, et al. Association of plasma phospholipid long-chain omega-3 fatty acids with incident atrial fibrillation in older adults: the Cardiovascular Health Study. *Circulation* 2012 Jan 26. [Epub ahead of print]

Zhu QQ, Lou DJ, Si XW, et al. Serum omega-3 polyunsaturated fatty acid and insulin resistance in type 2 diabetes mellitus and non-alcoholic fatty liver disease. *Zhonghua Nei Ke Za Zhi* 2010 Apr;49(4):305–308.

Chapter 19

Akihisa T, Tokuda H, Ogata M, et al. Cancer chemopreventive effects of polyunsaturated fatty acids. *Cancer Lett* 2004;205:9–13.

Alfano CM, et al. Fatigue, inflammation, and ?-3 and ?-6 fatty acid intake among breast cancer survivors. *J Clin Oncol* 2012 Mar 12. [Epub ahead of print]

American Cancer Society. Cancer facts and figures 2012. Atlanta: American Cancer Society, 2012. Available online at: www.cancer.org/acs/groups/content/@epidemiologysurvei-lance/documents/document/acspc-031941.pdf.

Bougnoux P, Hajjaji N, Ferrasson MN, et al., Improving outcome of chemotherapy of metastatic breast cancer by docosahexaenoic acid: a phase II trial. *Br J Cancer* 2009;101:1978–1985.

Brasky TM, Lampe JW, Potter JD, et al. Specialty supplements and breast cancer risk in the VITamins And Lifestyle (VITAL) cohort. *Cancer Epidemiol Biomarkers Prev* 2010;19(7): 1696–1708.

Brasky TM, Till C, White E, et al. Serum phospholipid fatty acids and prostate cancer risk: results from the Prostate Cancer Prevention Trial. *Am J Epidemiol* 2011 Jun 15;173(12):1429-1439.

Courtney ED, Matthews S, Finlayson C, et al. Eicosapentaenoic acid (EPA) reduces crypt cell proliferation and increases apoptosis in normal colonic mucosa in subjects with a history of colorectal adenomas. *Int. J. Colorectal Dis* 2007;22:765–776.

Fradet V, Cheng I, Casey G, et al. Dietary omega-3 fatty acids, cyclooxygenase-2 genetic variation, and aggressive prostate cancer risk. *Clin Cancer Res* 2009;15:2559–2566.

Gleissman H, Johnson JI, Kogner P. Omega-3 fatty acids in cancer: the protectors of good and the killers of evil? *Exp Cell Res* 2010;316(8):1365–1373.

Iigo M, Nakagawa T, Ishikawa C, et al. Inhibitory effects of docosahexaenoic acid on colon carcinoma 26 metastasis to the lung. *Br J Cancer* 1997;75:650–655.

Kelavkar UP, Hutzley J, Dhir R, et al. Prostate tumor growth and recurrence can be modulated by the omega-6: omega-3 ratio in diet: athymic mouse xenograft model simulating radical prostatectomy. *Neoplasia* 2006;8:112–124.

Kim J, Lim SY, Shin A, et al. Fatty fish and fish omega-3 fatty acid intakes decrease the breast cancer risk: a case-control study. *BMC Cancer* 2009 Jun 30;9:216.

Lanier AP, Holck P, Ehrsam Day G, et al. Childhood cancer among Alaska Natives. *Pediatrics* 2003;112:e396.

Leah E. Cancer cells: why DHA is not protectin. *Lipidomics Gateway* 2010 Mar 24. Available online at: www.lipidmaps.org/update/2010/100401/full/lipidmaps.2010.10.html.

Lindskog M, Gleissman H, Ponthan F, et al. Neuroblastoma cell death in response to docosahexaenoic acid: sensitization to chemotherapy and arsenic-induced oxidative stress. *Int I Cancer* 2006 May 15;118(10):2584–2593.

Manna S, Chakraborty T, Ghosh B, et al. Dietary fish oil associated with increased apoptosis and modulated expression of Bax and Bcl-2 during 7,12-dimethylbenz(alpha) anthracene-induced mammary carcinogenesis in rats. *Prostaglandins Leukot Essent Fatty Acids* 2008;79:5–14.

Noguchi M, Minami M, Yagasaki R, et al. Chemoprevention of DMBA-induced mammary carcinogenesis in rats by low-dose EPA and DHA. *Br J Cancer* 1997;75:348–353.

Noguchi M, Rose DP, Earashi M, et al. The role of fatty acids and eicosanoid synthesis inhibitors in breast carcinoma. *Oncology* 1995;52(4):265–271.

Norwegian Scientific Committee for Food Safety. Evaluation of negative and positive health effects of n-3 fatty acids as constituents of food supplements and fortified foods. 2011 Jun 28. Available online at: english.vkm.no/eway/default.aspx?pid=278&trg=Content_6424&Main_6359=6424:0:&Content_6424=6393:1861663::0:6425:1:::0:0.

Ramos EJ, Middleton FA, Laviano A, et al. Effects of omega-3 fatty acid supplementation on tumor-bearing rats. *J Am Coll Surg* 2004;199:716–723.

Smith-Warner SA, Spiegelman D, Ritz J, et al. Methods for pooling results of epidemiologic studies: the pooling project of prospective studies of diet and cancer. *Am J Epidemiol* 2006;163(11):1053–1064.

Szymanski KM, Wheeler DC, Mucci LA. Fish consumption and prostate cancer risk: a review and meta-analysis. *Am J Clin Nutr* 2010 Nov;92(5):1223–1233.

Takahashi M, Minamoto T, Yamashita N, et al. Reduction in formation and growth of 1, 2-dimethylhydrazine-induced aberrant crypt foci in rat colon by docosahexaenoic acid. *Cancer Res* 1993;53:2786–2789.

Thiebaut AC, Chajes V, Gerber M, et al. Dietary intakes of omega-6 and omega-3 poly-unsaturated fatty acids and the risk of breast cancer. *Int J Cancer* 2009;124:924–931.

Toriyama-Baba H, Iigo M, Asamoto M, et al. Organotropic chemopreventive effects of n-3 unsaturated fatty acids in a rat multi-organ carcinogenesis model. *Jpn J Cancer Res* 2001;92: 1175–1183.

Touvier M, et al. Modulation of the association between plasma intercellular adhesion molecule-1 and cancer risk by n-3 PUFA intake: a nested case-control study. *Am J Clin Nutr 2012* Apr;95(4):944–950.

van der Meij BS, et al. Oral nutritional supplements containing n-3 polyunsaturated fatty acids affect quality of life and functional status in lung cancer patients during multimo-dality treatment: an RCT. *Eur J Clin Nutr* 2012 Mar;66(3):399–404.

Williams CD, Whitley BM, Hoyo C, et al. A high ratio of dietary n-6/n-3 polyunsaturated fatty acids is associated with increased risk of prostate cancer. *Nutr Res* 2011;31(1):1-8).

Wolk A, Larsson SC, Johansson JE, et al. Long-term fatty fish consumption and renal cell carcinoma incidence in women. *JAMA* 2006;296:1371–1376.

Yuri T, Danbara N, Tsujita-Kyutoku M, et al. Dietary docosahexaenoic acid suppresses N-methyl-N-nitrosourea-induced mammary carcinogenesis in rats more effectively than eicosapentaenoic acid. *Nutr Cancer* 2003;45:211–217.

Chapter 20

Arterburn LM, Hall EB, Oken H. Distribution, interconversion, and dose response of n-3 fatty acids in humans. *Am J Clin Nutr* 2006 Jun;83(6 Suppl):1467S-1476S.

Dyerberg J, Madsen P, Møller JM, et al. Bioavailability of marine n-3 fatty acid formu-lations. *Prostaglandins Leukot Essent Fatty Acids* 2010;83:137–141.

Harris WS, Mozaffarian D, Lefevre M, et al. Towards establishing dietary reference intakes for eicosapentaenoic and docosahexaenoic acids. *J Nutr* 2009; 139(4):804S–819S.

Institute of Medicine. Dietary reference intakes for energy, carbohydrate, fiber, fat, fatty acids, cholesterol, protein, and amino acids. Washington, DC: National Academy Press, 2002/2005.

Index

Arachidonic acid (AA), 28, 32–33, 35, 38, 42, 50, 52, 56, 127, 181, 189, 200
Arrhythmias, 106
  atrial, 107–109
  ventricular, 109–111
Arteries, 35, 44, 84, 213
  narrowing of, 97, 99, 101–105
  stiffness, 104
Arteriosclerosis, 81
Arthritis, 44, 79, 102–103, 193–202
  osteo- , 195–196
  pain relief, 199–201
  reduction of medications for, 198–199
  rheumatoid, 194, 195, 196–197
  women and, 196, 197
Aspirin, 118
Asthma, 230
Atherosclerosis, 44, 82, 84, 97, 98–99, 101–102, 154
Athletes, 158–159, 200–201

Baked goods, processed, 179
Bang, Hans Olaf (H.O.), 4, 5, 74, 75
Beta-amyloid, 144–145
Bilateral drusen, 182
Biochemical individuality, 80
Bishop, Katherine Scott, 47
Bleeding, risk of, 35–36, 100, 115, 237
Block, R. C., 89
Blood, 26
  clots and clotting, 32, 33, 35, 40, 84, 98–101, 113, 114
  viscosity, 72
Blood pressure, 111, 114–115
Blue Mountains Eye Study, 180
Body, human, 19, 21
Bonds, 17
  cis, 23, 24
  double, 22–25, 29–30, 38
  location of, 25
  trans, 24
Brain, 25, 39, 44, 113, 125–132, 133–139
  volume, 146–147
Breastfeeding, 127, 128–129

Burping, 236
Burr, George Oswald, 47–49, 50, 191
Burr, Mildred Lawson, 48–49, 191

C-reactive protein (CRP), 42, 44–45, 103, 200, 226
Canadian Study of Health and Aging (CHSA), 149–150
Cancer, 41, 217–227, 231
  brain, 224–225
  breast, 219, 220–222, 225–226
  prostate, 220, 227
Carbohydrates, 204
Carbon, 14, 15–17, 19
  omega, 25
  omega-3, 25
Carboxyl terminal, 16, 19
Cardiovascular disease (CVD), 82, 83
Cardiovascular Heart Study, 108–109, 146
Cells, 133, 207, 217–218
  aging of, 86, 187–188
  foam, 99
  homeostatis, 59, 99
  membranes, 19, 21, 23, 24, 25–26, 30, 50, 58–60, 65, 106, 125, 186
  photoreceptor, 177–178
Centers for Disease Control and Prevention (CDC), 203, 205

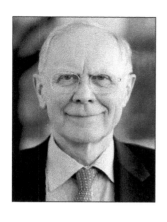

About the Authors

Jørn Dyerberg, M.D., DMSc., Hon. DMSc., is one of the world's leading authorities on the health benefits of omega-3 fish oils. He received his degree in medicine from the University of Aarhus in Aarhus, Denmark.

In 1971 Dr. Dyerberg published a landmark study in *The Lancet* regarding heart heath. In the early 1970s, he led a research team together with Dr. Bang that studied blood lipid levels among the Inuit population in Greenland. The group set out to find why the Inuit society had a low occurrence of heart disease, despite a diet of mostly seal and fish. Dr. Dyerberg first hypothesized that it was related to the abundance of the omega-3 fatty acids DHA and EPA in the fish. He eventually led five separate scientific expeditions to northwest Greenland to examine the association between omega-3, long-chain polyunsaturated fatty acid intake and coronary heart disease. Dr. Dyerberg has received several awards and accolades for this groundbreaking omega-3 research.

Dr. Dyerberg has held several physician positions at Denmark hospitals and research institutions, and since 2001 he has also served as a professor at the University of Copenhagen in Denmark. He is currently the medical and scientific advisor for Marine Ingredients in Mt. Bethel, Pennsylvania and Unilabs Ltd in Denmark.

His own research encompasses more than 350 scientific publications primarily concerning blood lipids, atherosclerosis, the blood coagulation system, omega-3 polyunsaturated fatty acids, trans fatty acids, and prostaglandins. His 1986 article in *Nutrition Reviews* on "Linolenate-derived polyunsaturated fatty acids and prevention of atherosclerosis" is among the top twenty most highly cited articles in the journal's seventy-year history.

In 2007 Dr. Dyerberg was honored by the American Heart Association in "Recognition of Outstanding Scientific Contribution for the Advancement of Heart Health Worldwide." In 2008, he received the American Dietetic Association Foundation's Edna and Robert Langholtz International Nutrition Award.

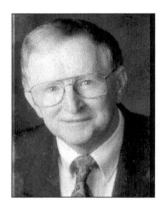

Richard A. Passwater, Ph.D., a research biochemist since 1959, is Director of Research for the Selenium Nutritional Research Center in Berlin, Maryland. He has written more than forty-five books and over 500 articles on nutrition. His laboratory research led to his discovery of biological antioxidant synergism in 1962 that has been the focus of his research and patents ever since. Dr. Passwater's research with selenium and other antioxidant nutrients has led to a series of patents relating to free radical pathology and health.

His 1982 book *EPA: Marine Lipids* (Keats Publishing) was the first book on fish oil and marine lipids and its wide distribution is credited with popularizing fish oil supplements with the public. In 1987, Dr. Passwater published *Fish Oil Update* (Keats Publishing), which went beyond the "why Eskimos don't get heart disease" story to discuss the expanding research into additional health roles including arthritis, lupus, and brain health. His books have been translated into eleven languages; Chinese, Spanish, French, German, Dutch, Japanese, Italian, Portuguese, Hebrew, Russian, and Swedish. Dr. Passwater is the scientific editor for *Whole Foods,* for which he writes the monthly column "Vitamin Connection" to help bring the latest research on nutrients to the public.

Dr. Passwater's discoveries have led to worldwide recognition. He was presented with the nutrition industry's Achievement Award for 1989 and the National Nutritional Foods Association's Presidents Award in 1999.

In 2004, he was awarded the James Lind Scientific Achievement Award and the John Peter Zenger Free Press Award for writing. Twice he has been honored by the Committee For World Health (1978 and 1980), and is listed in *Who's Who in the World*, *Who's Who in America*, *American Men and Women of Science*, and *Who's Who in the Frontiers of Science*.

www.ingramcontent.com/pod-product-compliance
Lightning Source LLC
Jackson TN
JSHW011356130125
77033JS00023B/707